医学英语新医科课程群系列教材

医学英语口语突破：朗读与复述

Medical English Breakthrough: Reading Aloud and Retelling

主 编 张 颖 曹 华

副主编 李 娜 饶 辉 符 莹

南京大学出版社

图书在版编目(CIP)数据

医学英语口语突破：朗读与复述 / 张颖，曹华主编.
— 南京：南京大学出版社，2021.7
ISBN 978 - 7 - 305 - 23495 - 8

Ⅰ. ①医… Ⅱ. ①张… ②曹… Ⅲ. ①医学－英语－
口语－医学院校－教材 Ⅳ. ①R

中国版本图书馆 CIP 数据核字(2020)第 109928 号

出版发行　南京大学出版社
社　　址　南京市汉口路 22 号　　　　邮　编　210093
出 版 人　金鑫荣
书　　名　**医学英语口语突破：朗读与复述**
主　　编　张 颖　曹 华
责任编辑　裴维维　　　　　　　　编辑热线　025 - 83592123
照　　排　南京南琳图文制作有限公司
印　　刷　南京京新印刷有限公司
开　　本　787×960　1/16　印张 11.25　字数 230 千
版　　次　2021 年 7 月第 1 版　2021 年 7 月第 1 次印刷
ISBN 978 - 7 - 305 - 23495 - 8
定　　价　37.00 元

网址：http://www.njupco.com
官方微博：http://weibo.com/njupco
官方微信号：njupress
销售咨询热线：(025) 83594756

前　言

随着国家不断加快对外开放的步伐，以英语为媒介的专业交流越来越普遍，专门用途英语的口头表达能力成为大学生的必备能力之一。《大学英语教学指南》(2020 版)明确要求大学英语"应进一步增强其学术英语或职业英语交流能力"。因此，医学院校的大学英语教学应当致力于培养医科学生以英语为媒介的专业交流能力。

编写目的

编写本书的目的是帮助医学专业的学习者提高语音、朗读和复述的能力与技巧，为更高阶段的学习打下坚实的基础。本书适用于在校医学生及其他中高级水平的英语学习者。

编写思路

不同于通用的口语教材，本书选材贴近医学专业学生的兴趣，适合就医学内容进行英语口语操练，提高英语口语能力。教程遵循"输出驱动，整合教学"的外语教学理念，语言输入与输出相结合，强调全球化背景下医学专业学习者英语表达与交流能力的培养；在帮助学习者提升英语语音与朗读复述技巧的同时，感受人文关怀，拓展知识视野，陶冶情操。

主要编写内容

教程由十个单元组成，每个单元包含两个板块：阅读复述和语音训练。

1. 阅读复述部分有两篇文章，选取简明通识的医学人文、医学文化、医学教育等方面的最新资料为素材。各单元文章编排语言由易到难，文意逐步加深，通过设计问答、概括文章、构建脑图、口头复述等灵活多样的训练形式，逐步提高学习者的口头表达能力。

2. 语音训练部分结合本单元文章语句，就不同英语语音及朗读技巧提供专项练习。配有英美籍人士录音。

本教程可以用于医学院校基础阶段英语课堂教学，教师可根据实际需要组织课堂活动，或采用翻转课堂形式组织教学。本教程也可作为听说课的补充教程或自主学习教程。

Contents
目　　录

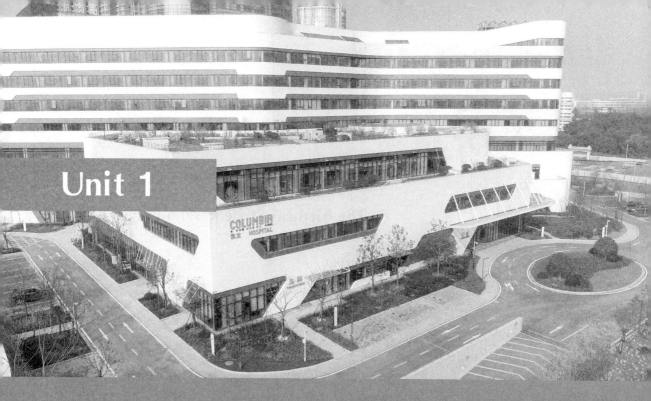

Unit 1

Upon completion of this unit，you will be able to：

- identify key plots in a narration
- retell the story with the help of connectives given
- learn the pronunciation skill of rising tone

✓音视频资源
✓参考答案
✓交流探讨

Text A

The Medical Student Who Cries

By Orly Farber

default [dɪ'fɔːlt] *n*. 默认；系统设定值

I'm a **default** crier. I happy-cry, stress-cry, romantic-comedy-cry, regular-comedy-cry and, apparently, I even doctor-in-training-cry.

Crying is a tough response, especially for someone who wants to take care of sick patients. My default reaction poses challenges for my future career. I had my first taste of this when a patient actor brought me to tears. An actor? That's ridiculous, you might think. It was all pretend and yet, I broke down. I'm a soft person, but it wasn't a soft cry. I'm talking deep **heaves**, **snot** running, **mascara smeared** on my glasses.

heave [hiːv] *n*. 举；拖；拉；抛；起伏
snot [snɒt] *n*. 鼻涕
mascara [mæ'skɑːrə] *n*. 睫毛膏；染睫毛油
smear [smɪə(r)] *v*. 胡乱涂抹；弄脏
pick on 跟……找碴；故意刁难

The actor's role was to be a difficult patient, to **pick on** first-year medical students and throw us off our recently established clinical game. I was prepared. I had read the assigned articles about redirecting "difficult patient encounters" and had gotten a good night's sleep.

"Oh jeez, not another woman," the patient said as I entered.

"Hi, are you Mr. Jones?" I asked in my friendly,

tempered clinical tone.

"Are you the doctor?" he spat.

"No，I'm Orly Farber. I'm a first-year medical student and part of your care team—"

"You're a medical student!" he interrupted，"And a woman? I want to see the real doctor. A male doctor！"

And so it went.

For a few minutes，I handled the case with about as much **professionalism** and **composure** as I could **muster**. I told him he could see the doctor after I collected some more information，but I couldn't promise that the doctor would be a man. He got **agitated**，raised his voice，and refused to answer my questions. I stayed calm. Then he pointed to my shoes.

"Look at you," he **sneered**，"wearing your stupid shiny penny **loafers**. You've probably never experienced a day of struggle in your life. How could you possibly understand my pain?"

"Sir，I wouldn't make any assumptions," I replied **sternly**,"I'm just here to listen and learn about your pain ..." My voice **quivered**，the **prodrome** to my tears.

I turned to the advisor observing me and asked for a timeout；she nodded. I looked at my classmates，who were also watching the encounter，their eyebrows raised to the ceiling. "How's it going?" my advisor said，"Are you feeling OK?"

---

temper［'tempə(r)］*v.* 使缓和；使温和

professionalism ［prə'feʃnəlɪzəm］*n.* 专业水平；专业素质

composure［kəm'pəʊʒə(r)］*n.* 沉着；镇静；镇定

muster［'mʌstə(r)］*v.* 找寻；聚集；激起(支持、勇气等)

agitate［'ædʒɪteɪt］*v.* 激怒

sneer［snɪə(r)］*v.* 嘲笑；讥讽

loafer［'ləʊfə(r)］*n.* 乐福鞋；平底便鞋

sternly［'stɜːnlɪ］*adv.* 严厉地；严肃地

quiver［'kwɪvə(r)］*v.* 轻微颤动；抖动

prodrome［'prəʊdrəʊm］*n.* 前驱症状；先兆

feedback loop ['fiːdbæk luːp]
反馈环路；反馈回路

empathize ['empəθaɪz] v.
有同感；产生共鸣；表同情

grievance ['griːvəns] n.
不平的事；委屈；抱怨；牢
骚

stoically adv. 坚忍地

And like every time someone asks if I'm OK，like after tripping in public or receiving some bad news，I cracked. Hard.

For me，crying is a positive **feedback loop**：I cry because I'm sad or stressed or scared. And then，after a few seconds，I cry because I'm crying—because I'm embarrassed or feel weak or wish I could respond in any other way.

That day，I cried because a patient actor yelled at me. He challenged my place in medicine as a woman and more so，he doubted my ability to **empathize**，a trait I proudly wear on my sleeve. And then，when the initial tears had been shed，I cried out of shame，for having lost my cool in public，in front of my classmates and professors，in front of an actor with fake **grievances**.

I don't yet know how to manage my emotionality in a clinical space. I want to be soft，but not too soft. I want to maintain my compassion，without losing my composure. And so I hope that going forward I learn how to handle my tears，not just how to redirect a "difficult encounter," but how to redirect my own reactions. I hope that the next time a patient insults my favorite penny loafers or questions my place in medicine and my expertise，I won't burst into tears. Instead，I'll **stoically** face him and say，"Sir，these loafers have saved lives."

Task 1

Come up with 6 questions about the text. The questions can be about the main idea or important details of the text. They can also be inference drawn from the text or lessons learned.

Model question:

1. What do you learn about the author's personality from the text?

2. _____

3. _____

4. _____

5. _____

6. _____

Task 2

Answer the questions in Task 1.

1. What do you learn about the author's personality from the text?

_____

_____

_____

_____

_____

_____

2. _____

_____

_____

_____

_____

3. _____

_____

_____

_____

_____

4. _____

_____

_____

_____

_____

5. _____

_____

_____

_____

_____

6. _____

_____

_____

_____

_____

Task 3

Retell the story of the author's clinical role play in your own words. Please use third person narration instead of first person. The following connectives are for your reference.

before	when	so	but	because
however	then	after	finally	

Text B

Why I Study Memory

By Wendy Suzuki, PhD

Long before I ever wanted to be a **neuroscientist**, I wanted to be a Broadway star. But despite my early **showbiz** dreams, I quickly and easily fell into a life of total science **geekdom**, and I followed those scientific **aspirations** to the University of California, Berkeley, my family's **Alma Mater**.

neuroscientist
[ˈnjʊroʊˌsaɪəntɪst] *n.* 神经
科学家;神经学家
showbiz [ˈʃəʊbɪz] *n.* 同
show business;娱乐行业;
娱乐界;演艺界
geekdom [giːkdəm] *n.*
the state of being a geek
aspiration [ˌæspəˈreɪʃn]
n. 渴望;抱负;志向
Alma Mater [ˈælməˈmɑːtə
(r)] *n.* 母校

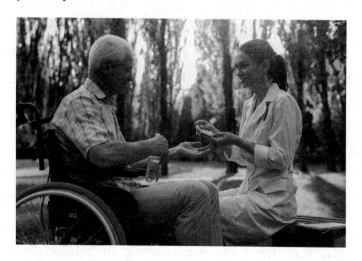

Now, you have to understand, I come from a very serious Japanese American family. We are always pleasant and very polite but never overly **affectionate**. You can think of us as a Japanese American version of

affectionate [əˈfekʃənət]
a. 充满深情的;满怀柔情
的;表示爱的

Downton Abbey, without the accent, the servants, or the real estate. That's us. So when the time came, Mom and Dad packed me up in the car and drove me there, and again, Downton Abbey: We didn't hug. We just waved goodbye.

Soon after arriving at the university, I found the perfect outlet for my science geekiness: a class called The Brain and Its Potential, taught by Professor Marian Diamond. On the first day of class, she slowly opened the lid of the hatbox she had brought and very carefully pulled out a real human brain, the first one I had ever seen.

She told us that what she was holding in her hands was the most complex structure known to humankind; it defined our personalities and creativity and allowed us to go from laughing to crying from one second to the next. She said that one of the most amazing things about the brain is that it can change in response to the environment, a trait called brain **plasticity**. It was at that moment I realized I wanted to be a neuroscientist.

For my career in neuroscience, I studied a form of everyday brain plasticity: long-term memory. I became an expert in the **anatomy**, **physiology**, and function of the brain areas important for long-term memory, fascinated with how a single experience could live on in our brains for 60, 70, or even 80 years.

But one day after I had started my own research lab at New York University, a particularly **poignant**

plasticity [plæ'stɪsətɪ] n. 可塑性

anatomy [ə'nætəmɪ] n. 解剖学
physiology [ˌfɪzi'ɒlədʒɪ] n. 生理学

poignant ['pɔɪnjənt] adj. 令人沉痛的；悲惨的；酸楚的

newspaper article about the bond between a father and son made me realize that despite the fact that I was a memory expert, I spent very little time thinking about the personal aspects of memory—that is, how precious our memories are and how they define us.

Sometime after I read that article, my mother called to tell me that Dad wasn't feeling well. Not only that, she said he couldn't remember how to drive to the 7-eleven where he had bought his morning coffee for the past 30 years.

Now, that was scary. I jumped into action and called my colleagues at Stanford University to find him the best **neurologist** I could. Dad got better, but his memory didn't recover.

neurologist [njʊəˈrɒlədʒɪst]
n. 神经病学家；神经科医生

Me, I just felt guilty. What good was being an expert on memory if I couldn't do one little thing to help my father get his memory back?

As I had gotten older, my relationship with my parents had grown closer, and I would call them every Sunday to chat. But after my Dad's memory problem developed, I knew I wanted to start to shift our relationship in a new direction.

While there was never any question that my parents loved my brother and me, the fact was, we never said "I love you" to each other as adults. I decided that I wanted to start saying those words to my parents. But because we had never said it before, I couldn't just start saying it to them out of the blue. I would have to ask permission.

I was feeling uncomfortable about making this call，but I realized it wasn't because of the awkwardness of making the request. It was because I was afraid they might say no.

But there was only one way to know their answer，so one Sunday，I gathered up all my courage and called. My theme that night was "Keep it light". I said，"How you doing? Here's my week. How was your week?" And sometime during the conversation，I said，"hey，Mom. You know，we never say 'I love you.' What do you think about the idea of starting to say that when we talk to each other?"

There was a long silence on the phone，and my stomach went all the way up to my throat. Then she said，"I think that's a great idea." Thank goodness she said yes! I said to myself. But keeping with my theme，I said，"That's great!" and we continued our conversation.

Then the tension started rising again. It's one thing to agree to say "I love you," but it's another thing to actually say it.

It had been my request，so I **took the bull by the horns**. I said，"Okayyy—in other words，get ready，Mom. I love you!" And she said，"I love you too!" And we had done it.

Then it was Dad's turn. I knew because I made it

take the bull by the horns
勇敢面对危险或困境

through with Mom，Dad would be easy. So I asked my Dad. He said yes. We said our awkward "I love you," and the night of the Big Ask was over.

I was **triumphant**，but as soon as I got off the phone，I broke down in tears. Not only had I said "I love you" to my parents for the first time as an adult，I realized that night，I had changed the culture of our family. Forever.

triumphant［traɪˈʌmfənt］ *adj.* 高奏凯歌的；大获全胜的；扬扬得意的

The next week，I called as usual，and you'll be happy to know that my "I love you" with my Mom was much less awkward. Then it was time to talk to Dad.

I realized that he might not remember we had made this agreement last week，so I was ready to remind him. But that night，he surprised me. Because that night and every Sunday since，he has said "I love you" first.

Now，you have to remember that sometimes my Dad can't quite remember whether I'm visiting for Thanksgiving or Christmas. But somehow，he was able to make this memory stick.

And I know why. As a neuroscientist，I know that emotional **resonance** helps us remember.

resonance［ˈrezənəns］ *n.* 共鸣；共振

So the love or maybe even the pride he felt because his daughter asked whether she could say "I love you" to him—it beat **dementia** and allowed him to form a new long-term memory. And you can be sure that I will keep that memory for the rest of my life.

dementia［dɪˈmenʃə］ *n.* 痴呆；精神错乱

And now that is why I study memory.

Task 1

Come up with 10 questions about the text. The questions can be about the main idea or important details of the story. They can also be inference drawn from the text or lessons learned.

Model question：

1. Why does the author mention Downton Abbey in Paragraph 2?

2. _____

3. _____

4. _____

5. _____

6. _____

7. _____

8. _____

9. _____

10. _____

Task 2

Answer the questions in Task 1.

Model question & answer：

1. Why does the author mention Downton Abbey in Paragraph 2?

Answer：The author, from a Japanese American family, makes an analogy between Downton Abbey and her family. They both have serious atmosphere. The author's family members are always pleasant and very polite but never overly affectionate. Even when the author left home for university, which is a significant event, parents and daughter didn't hug like average American families. They just waved goodbye.

2. _____

3. _____

4. _____

5. _____

6. _____

7. _____

8. _____

9. _____

10. _____

Task 3

1. Complete the following flow chart about the story.

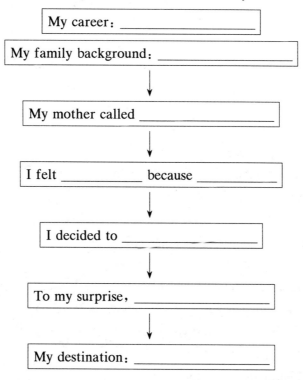

My career: _____

My family background: _____

↓

My mother called _____

↓

I felt _____ because _____

↓

I decided to _____

↓

To my surprise, _____

↓

My destination: _____

2. Choose the appropriate connectives from the box and retell the story based on the chart. (You don't have to use all of the connectives.)

when	so	a week later	because	however	then	after

Reading Aloud

A. 升调（rising tone）

英语中的升调一般用于：

1. 一般疑问句，如

Is there a stamp show on Sunday? ↗

Do you mind uncrossing your legs though? ↗

2. 选择疑问句的前半部分，如：

Is he an English teacher ↗ or French teacher? ↘

Are you here for the shoes ↗ or socks? ↘

3. 若干相同类目的词汇并列出现时（最后一项除外），如：

My ideal man must be handsome ↗, intelligent ↗, generous ↗ and considerate.

I wish you would appreciate that I have to orchestrate a complex network of 26 bones ↗, nearly three dozen joints ↗, and more than 100 muscles ↗, tendons ↗, and ligaments for every single step you take.

4. 表示疑问的陈述句，如：

You want a cup of tea? ↗

You feel that pain from ankle to inner arch? ↗

B. Read aloud after the recording.

1. "Hi, are you Mr. Jones ↗?" I asked in my friendly ↗, tempered ↗ clinical tone. ↘

2. My advisor said, "Are you feeling OK ↗?"

3. "You're a medical student!" he interrupted, "And a woman ↗? I want to see the real doctor. A male doctor!"

4. I happy-cry ↗, stress-cry ↗, romantic-comedy-cry ↗, regular-comedy-cry ↗ and, apparently, I even doctor-in-training-cry. ↘

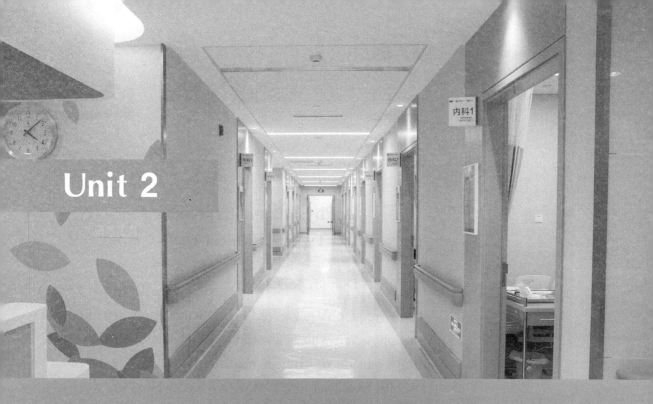

Unit 2

Upon completion of this unit , you will be able to：

- narrate actions in sequence of time
- draw a mind map to illustrate main points of a text
- summarize differences between 2 concepts
- summarize main points of a text
- learn the pronunciation skill of falling tone

✓音视频资源
✓参考答案
✓交流探讨

Text A

physician [fɪˈzɪʃn] n. 医师；(尤指)内科医生

entrepreneur [ˌɒntrəprəˈnɜː(r)] n. 创业者，企业家

A Physician-entrepreneur's Typical Clinical Day

By Suneel Dhand, MD

I frequently get asked how I balance my schedule as a physician who is also involved in lots of different things outside of clinical medicine. As any reader of my blog knows, I like to stay busy! As well as my work as a **frontline** physician (which I absolutely love and have no intention of ever leaving)—doing a mixture of **inpatient** and **outpatient** work, I also am involved in other ventures including **startup** work. I've always known from when I was in medical school that I had a creative side to me, that would seek other **outlets** for my ideas and energy levels. Every week is different, and I like to keep things interesting and varied—**striving** for zero chance of boredom! But at the same time, I've never believed that life is all about work, and was fortunately blessed with parents who encouraged me right from a very young age, to do lots of other things in my spare time, including traveling and getting outdoors to play sports.

I'm going to talk to you through my typical weekday schedule. While every day is different, I've

frontline [ˈfrʌntlaɪn] n. 前线

inpatient [ˈɪnpeɪʃnt] n. 住院病人

outpatient [ˈaʊtpeɪʃnt] n. 门诊病人

startup [ˈstɑːtʌp] n. 启动；新兴公司

outlet [ˈaʊtlet] n. (感情、思想、精力发泄的)出路；表现机会

strive [straɪv] v. 努力；奋斗；力争；力求

tried staying true to the broad schedule most of the time.

My daily schedule as a physician

4:30—5 a.m.: Wake up. I actually haven't always been a morning person, but have trained myself to become this way, based on what I've learned and read about the habits of the most successful people.

5—5:30 a.m.: **Confirm** my daily agenda and catch up on a few things from overnight. Browse through emails, read through the news quickly, and perhaps start writing something.

confirm [kən'fɜːm] v. 确认

5:30—6 a.m.: A quick workout, at least 20 minutes of **cardiovascular** with some weight training. I am not a big breakfast person, and will typically have a healthy cereal bar with a cup of tea (I do not drink coffee).

cardiovascular [ˌkɑːdɪəʊˈvæskjələ(r)] adj. 心血管的

6:30—7 a.m.: Arrive at the hospital and start rounding on patients. I like to get the day started as early as possible, because an hour in the morning is worth three at any other time of day.

7 a.m.—1 p.m.: See patients, get plans in place, **prioritizing** the sickest patients first. Usually, stop for a brief break around 10:30 a.m. to gather my thoughts, clear my mind, accompanied by a fresh juice or cup of tea (plus/minus another cereal bar depending on how hungry I am!).

prioritize [praɪˈɒrətaɪz] v. 按重要性排列;划分优先顺序;优先处理

1 p.m.: Catch up on emails and any other messages. Typically have a small healthy lunch, before getting right back to work.

discharge [dɪs'tʃɑːdʒ] v.
准许(某人)离开,出院

1—5 p. m.: Continue rounding on or **discharging** patients and admitting new ones via the Emergency room. See some patients a second time and usually have family meetings during this time as well. I have a to-do list that I create during my day, and as the afternoon progresses, check my way through these items. Tasks may include calling other doctors and chasing up results. Oh, and I usually always have a cup of Earl Grey tea around 4 p.m. (an English thing I guess).

5—5:30 p. m.: Aim to finish work in the hospital. Barring any emergency, I am not one to hang around very late in the evenings at work. I'd far rather start the day much earlier, so I can get home at a reasonable time.

6 p. m.: Fortunately, I've never lived far from where I work (did you know research shows that for every **increment** your commute is more than 30 minutes, your job dissatisfaction goes dramatically up?). When I get home, I may have a healthy snack such as an apple or banana.

increment ['ɪŋkrəmənt]
n. 增量;增加

6—7:30 p. m.: I will often exercise again for 30 minutes or so, either at the gym or go for a quick run, before showering and feeling fresh again after a long day. I will then catch up with my own (startup) work-related emails, write, and perform any other home-related errands quickly—like opening the mail, doing the washing.

7:30 p. m. +: I am pretty strict about having evenings to myself, and at least one complete day a week where I'm not working or going at 110% light speed!

Whether it's catching up with friends, going on a date, enjoying a Netflix show, Lindy Hop swing dancing (my latest hobby) or just doing nothing—this is my time! Phone and Internet away, please. Dinner is also around this time, but rarely after 8:30 p.m.

10 p.m.: Assuming I'm working in the hospital again the next day, I'll be in bed by this time. May have a real quick catch up on emails around this time. Oh, and I always try to read before going to bed. We all have our own **optimal** sleep amounts (studies suggest ideal sleep for most people is between 6 and 8 hours). For me, it's around 6.5 hours.

optimal [ˈɒptɪməl] *adj.*
最优的;最佳的

Task 1

Summarize how the author spends a typical weekday as a physician and an entrepreneur based on his schedule.

The doctor wakes up at 4:30 to 5 in the morning. After that _____

_____

_____

_____

_____

_____

_____

_____

Task 2

Come up with 6 questions about the text. The questions can be about the main idea or important details of the text. They can also be inference drawn from the text or lessons learned.

Model question：

1. What kind of life does the author live?

2. _____

3. _____

4. _____

5. _____

6. _____

Task 3

Answer the questions in Task 2.

1. What kind of life does the author live?

_____

_____

_____

_____

2. _____

_____

_____

_____

_____

3. _____

_____

_____

_____

_____

_____

4. _____

_____

_____

_____

_____

_____

5. _____

_____

_____

_____

_____

_____

6. _____

_____

_____

_____

_____

_____

Text B

compassionate
[kəm'pæʃənət] *adj.* 有同情心的；表示怜悯的

Compassionate Doctor-Patient Relationships

Interview with Dr. Hyla Cass

Interviewed by Lyle Hurd

Lyle Hurd：I'd like to welcome Dr. Hyla Cass back to our conversation. Dr. Cass，we've talked about your commitment to your being a woman on a mission，and your commitment to treating the whole person rather than just the symptoms. You have also an attitude toward the way the doctor patient relationship should be handled. When did you begin to really get involved in this whole concept ... that there's a real need for that kind of communication?

Dr. Hyla Cass：I'm so glad you asked. My ... first role model was my dad，who was a family physician practicing out of our home in Toronto. And from the earliest that I can remember，patients were coming to the house. I would answer the door，**usher** them in；he didn't have a big staff，it was just him and me. Well，at least I answered the door，I don't know if I was much help. But he was a great，great role model. He took me on calls，he would take me to the hospital，and I saw what a doctor did. I saw how he interacted with patients，how entire families would come in，how

usher ['ʌʃə(r)] *v.* 把……引往；引导；引领

he'd go to people's homes and see them in their natural environment, and how generous he was, and really, pretty **holistic**. He was treating people's lifestyle, he was treating the whole person, and he used minimal drugs. And I remember as new drugs would come out, and other doctors were using them, he would be warning patients to be really cautious, and rightly so. Let's wait awhile, that turned out to be not so good for people. So he had a very good **intuitive** sense about what to do, and passed that on to me. ... As I was growing up people asked me what I wanted to be when I grew up. I thought I was going to be a nurse to help my daddy, or actually be a doctor, and he really did encourage me to go to medical school. I think women who have **mentors** like that, who encourage them to do that—it's really wonderful, and I still appreciate his presence, and he continues to inspire me. He passed away 10 years ago; he's still a great inspiration to me.

LH: You know, that's pretty interesting. We today say, that basically, to have things work, first people have to be **co-captains** of their own health care team. Sounds to me like your dad made his patients ... participants on their own health care team.

HC: I think so. And I think that's [what] I'm encouraging people to do as well. There's no way, for example, someone comes in to me, and I've determined what supplements they need, [that] they [don't] still need to be pretty much in contact with me, regarding how these things are working. It's not

holistic [hə'lɪstɪk] *adj.*
整体的；全面的

intuitive [ɪn'tjuːɪtɪv] *adj.*
凭直觉得到的；直觉的

mentor ['mentɔː(r)] *n.*
导师；顾问

co-captain [ˌkəʊ'kæptɪn]
n. 副队长

prescription [prɪ'skrɪpʃn] *n*. 处方；药方

interactive [ˌɪntər'æktɪv] *adj*. 合作的；相互影响的；互动的

tremendous [trə'mendəs] *adj*. 巨大的；极大的

just here's a **prescription**, goodbye, see you in a month or two. It's send me an email. Give me a phone call. Let's talk about how you're doing. Add one new supplement at a time and fill in the food-mood journal, a food-mood supplement journal. Let's be very **interactive**. This will take a lot of my time, but it makes such a **tremendous** difference. They know that I'm there. They learn not to be too imposing on my time; I think it really works out very well. It's very much a mutual process and the results really show that.

LH：Thank you very much. It's nice to have you.

HC：A pleasure.

Task 1

Draw a mind map to illustrate why Dr. Hyla Cass's father was "a great role model" based on what you learn from the text.

Task 2

What are differences between treating the whole person and treating the symptoms? Fill in the following table to answer this question.

Treating the whole person	Treating the symptoms
Treating patients' lifestyle	
Encouraging patients and family members to get involved	
	Only communicate during visit
Very interactive	
	Not very time-consuming
Mutual process	

Task 3

With the help of previous tasks, summarize what compassionate doctor-patient relationships consist of.

Reading Aloud

A. 降调（falling tone）

英语中的降调一般用于：

1. 特殊疑问句：

How was your week? ↘

What do you think about the idea of going for a picnic? ↘

2. 感叹句：

What depressing information! ↘

How difficult the situation is! ↘

3. 反义疑问句，当说话人对自己所说的内容已经很确定，只是象征性地与对方确认一下时：

A small world, isn't it? ↘

You've heard about it, haven't you? ↘

4. 选择疑问句的最后一个选项，如：

Will you go there by bus ↗ or by train? ↘

Do you prefer hand-written letter ↗ or e-mail? ↘

5. 并列出现的若干相同类目词语的最后一项，如：

I became an expert in anatomy ↗, physiology ↗, and function of the brain areas. ↘

B. Read aloud after the recording.

1. Every week is different ↘, and I like to keep things interesting and varied ↘—striving for zero chance of boredom! ↘

2. Browse through emails ↗, read through the news quickly ↗, and perhaps start writing something. ↘

3. I saw how he interacted with patients ↗, how entire families would come in ↗, how he'd go to people's homes and see them in their natural environment ↗, and how generous he was, and really, pretty holistic. ↘

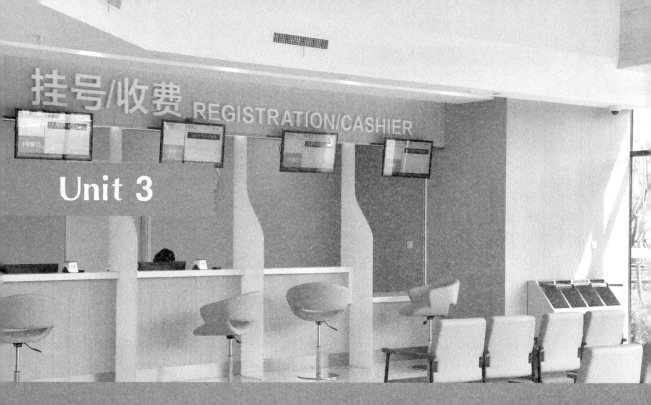

Unit 3

Upon completion of this unit，you will be able to：

- identify key plots by composing interview
- extract key words before answering questions
- analyze structure of narrative text
- draw a flow chart before narrating a procedure
- learn the rules of stressed and unstressed pronunciations

✓音视频资源
✓参考答案
✓交流探讨

Text A

empathy ['empəθɪ] n. 同感；共鸣；同情

innate [ɪ'neɪt] adj. 天生的；先天的；与生俱来的

open-ended [ˌəʊpən 'endɪd] adj. 无限制的；无确定目标的

interject [ˌɪntə'dʒekt] v. 打断(别人的讲话)；插话

foster ['fɒstə(r)] v. 促进；助长

acquire [ə'kwaɪə(r)] v. 获得；得到

rotation [rəʊ'teɪʃn] n. 轮换；交替；换班

impervious [ɪm'pɜːvɪəs] adj. 不受影响的

residency ['rezɪdənsɪ] n. 住院医生实习期

Can Empathy be Taught, or Is It Innate?

By Okechukwu Anochie, MD

In medical school, I was taught to sit down at eye-level when speaking to a patient, ask them how they'd prefer to be addressed, make sure to ask questions in an **open-ended** manner to allow patients to express themselves, and **interject** with "that must be really difficult for you" or "I can only imagine how that makes you feel," as a way to show empathy and **foster** better connection with patients during the interview process of **acquiring** the patient's history of present illness.

This worked for some patients during my medical school clinical **rotations**; however, I've seen some patients become **impervious** to such an approach, sometimes becoming upset or emotionally closed-off.

In **residency**, I've encountered many patients who do not respond to the empathic methods I was trained to use during the history-taking process. During these times, I've learned to abandon the script and speak to these patients from a perspective of dignity and respect and have rarely ever had trouble connecting even with the most "difficult" patient.

Some of my colleagues have asked me how being empathetic comes so naturally to me, or how did I learn to connect so well with my patients?

"Even the most **cantankerous**, **bellicose**, and unreasonable patients calm down and become agreeable after speaking with you!"

I'm not quite sure either. I see patients as people first.

They need to know you care; that you really value and respect them, despite meeting you at the most **vulnerable** and worst times of their life. That patient who gets admitted every two weeks like clockwork for alcohol withdrawal or **heroin overdose** needs to know that you, as a physician, still respect their dignity (however little it is). They need us to understand that their diseases or struggles do not define them as a person and that they have value in the eyes of their family and loved ones.

Questions such as: do you know why you're in the hospital? What do you think is your current **diagnosis** or what medical problem do you think you currently have that we're treating? What have we done for you so far? Have you seen all the labs and imaging results yet? Would you like me to explain them to you? What are you most concerned about right now? It doesn't have to be about the disease we're treating. Is there anything else I can do to help you or make you feel more comfortable? Is there somebody you'd like me to

cantankerous [kæn'tæŋkərəs] *adj.* 脾气坏且抱怨不休的

bellicose ['belɪkəus] *adj.* 好争辩的;好斗的;好战的

vulnerable ['vʌlnərəbl] *adj.* 脆弱的,易受……伤害的

heroin ['herəuɪn] *n.* 海洛因

overdose ['əuvədəus] *n.* (一次用药)过量

diagnosis [ˌdaɪəg'nəusɪs] *n.* 诊断

call on your behalf? By the way, my name is Dr. Anochie ("It's like Spanish for last night," if the patient is Hispanic). I'll do my best to take care of you.

These are simple conversations to have with patients, but they are also very meaningful to them. It informs the patients that you care about their understanding of their disease process, and that you're also providing emotional support to help them deal with it. They perceive you as their ally and **advocate**. Frequently checking in on patients **inadvertently** causes them to pull down their walls and trust you as their physician. This is essential because the physician-patient trust significantly increases **compliance** with recommendations, prescriptions, and clinic appointments after the inpatient discharge process.

advocate ['ædvəkeɪt] *n.* 拥护者；支持者
inadvertently [ˌɪnəd'vɜːtəntlɪ] *adv.* 无意地；不经意地
compliance [kəm'plaɪəns] *n.* 服从；顺从；遵从

This still begs the question: Can empathy be taught?

Can't I just memorize some sentences that project empathy and say them to a patient while holding their hands and staring into their eyes, and check it off my list?

It doesn't work that way.

Patients know when doctors are "acting."

It's like listening to customer service **rep** tell you "thank you so much for calling, we really value your **membership**," you know it's a memorized line spoken

rep [rep] *n.* 推销员；销售代表
membership ['membəʃɪp] *n.* 会员资格

perfunctorily. My personal belief is that empathy comes naturally to people who have had some background experience to draw from when attempting to connect with a patient.

A physician who's had friends or relatives suffer through drug addiction will easily know how to connect with a "**frequent flyer**" drug addict, etc. This **underscores** the importance of admitting students into medical schools with diverse personal life experiences, social-economic classes, and family **upbringing**. Future doctors from such varied backgrounds are vital to the field of medicine, and they will make a positive impact toward improving the health care experience for our diverse and complicated patient population.

A quote from the late Maya Angelou, "I've learned that people will forget what you said, people will forget what you did, but people will never forget how you made them feel," perfectly **encapsulates** the theme of this opinion piece.

It is also common knowledge that empathetic physicians are less likely to get a **malpractice** lawsuit even after admitting an error or mistake to a patient or their family. It is also important to acknowledge that we, as physicians, also learn from our patients' stories and experiences beyond their presenting chief complaint or working diagnosis. I've learned so much from the diverse patient population I care for.

I've gone home in tears, sometimes thinking about

perfunctorily [pə'fʌŋktərɪlɪ] *adv*. 敷衍地；马马虎虎

frequent flyer [ˌfriːkwənt 'flaɪə(r)] 飞行常客；常客

underscore [ˌʌndə'skɔː(r)] *v*. 在……下面划线；强调；着重说明

upbringing ['ʌpbrɪŋɪŋ] *n*. 抚育；养育；教养；培养

encapsulate [ɪn'kæpsjʊleɪt] *v*. 简述；概括；压缩

malpractice [ˌmæl'præktɪs] *n*. 渎职；玩忽职守

regale [rɪ'geɪl] v. (以故事或笑话)极力取悦

persevere [ˌpɜːsə'vɪə(r)] v. 坚持；孜孜以求

preferential [ˌprefə'renʃl] adj. 优先的；优惠的；优待的

how the health care system is failing them. I've also been inspired when patients voluntarily share their personal triumphs, **regaling** how they've overcome impossible circumstances, and are still **persevering** to get through the next day. This is why I love medicine. This is also why I advocate for my patients and treat everyone with equal dignity, whether they're a drug addict or CEO of a Fortune 500 company. Death and disease do not respect class or age; neither should physicians give **preferential** treatments to them.

Task 1

Suppose there is a TV interview with the author of this article about empathy in clinical circumstance. What questions would you ask if you were the interviewer? How would you answer them if you were the interviewee?

Question: Hello, Dr. Anochie. You do a great job in connecting with patients. So I wonder if you learn that from medical school.

Answer: Well, I did learn a lot from medical school. _____

But _____

_____

Q: _____

A: _____

_____

Q: _____

A: _____

_____

Q: _____
A: _____

_____

_____

Q: _____
A: _____

_____

_____

Q: _____
A: _____

_____

_____

Task 2

How do you answer the question in the title: "Can empathy be taught, or is it innate?"

1. Before answering this question, list the key points that you use to support you answer.

2. Now answer the question in a short passage, based on the key points you listed.

Text B

trucker [ˈtrʌkə(r)] *n.* 卡车司机

dusk [dʌsk] *n.* 黄昏；暮色

general-surgery intern 普外科实习生

on call 随时待命的

fatigue [fəˈtiːg] *n.* 疲劳；劳累

snap [snæp] *v.* 打开

hum [hʌm] *n.* 嗡嗡声；嘈杂声

blacktop [ˈblæktɒp] *n.* （铺路面用的）柏油碎石

eerie [ˈɪərɪ] *adj.* 怪异的；神秘的

blink back 尽力用眨眼来控制

weave [wiːv] *v.* 编，织

lanky [ˈlæŋki] *adj.* 瘦长（或胳膊、腿细长）而行动笨拙的

cab [kæb] *n.* 驾驶室

honk [hɒŋk] *v.* （使汽车喇叭）鸣响

A Trucker, a Doctor, and a Lifesaving Coincidence

By Maxine Rock

Dusk had descended quickly, and Sherry Apple knew she was in danger. Apple, a 34-year-old **general-surgery intern**, had been **on call** at Georgia Baptist Medical Center in Atlanta (now Atlanta Medical Center) for more than two days, with only a few hours' sleep. And now **fatigue** was clouding her eyes as she drove to a meeting in Louisville, Kentucky, nearly seven hours away.

She tried **snapping** on her CB radio, which truckers and enthusiasts used to chat and warn one another about road conditions, but the airwaves were silent. Soon the **hum** of the tires on the **blacktop** became an **eerie** lullaby, and Apple was **blinking back** drowsiness. Her car started to **weave**.

A **lanky** 41-year-old trucker named Woody Key was in the **cab** of his 18-wheeler when his headlights picked up a silver sports car ahead, drifting out of its lane. Key **honked** his horn and yelled into his CB microphone, "Four-wheeler, are you all right?" His lights outlined a blonde in the driver's seat, her head bent forward. "Wake up, lady!" he screamed. "Wake up!"

Apple snapped to attention, her heart pounding. She picked up the CB mike. "I'm exhausted, and I'm lucky I'm still alive driving this tired. Thanks!"

"Call me Woodpecker, my CB handle," the trucker said. "I'm goin' to Kentucky. And you?"

"Kentucky."

"Well, good! I'll travel behind and help keep you awake. What's your handle?"

"Dr. Froot Loops," she told him. When he laughed, she explained that that was what the kids on the **pediatric** ward had called her.

pediatric [ˌpiːdɪˈætrɪk] *adj*. 小儿科的

As the long miles unfolded, they swapped stories and jokes, and the time passed quickly. Woodpecker and Dr. Froot Loops parted near the Kentucky state line. She thanked him for keeping her awake and safe on the long, dark road. "I enjoyed the talk," he said. The truck **rumbled** past, and the alert, considerate stranger was gone.

rumble['rʌmbl] *v*. 发出持续而低沉的声音

Some time later, on November 22, 1986, a **trauma** alert **blared** from the Georgia Baptist Medical Center loudspeaker. Apple entered the trauma unit and found several surgeons bending over the bloody form of an accident victim brought in from a two-truck collision. Both arms and legs were broken. His **rib cage** was crushed. His face had been smashed. Worst of all,

trauma ['trɔːmə] *n*. 损伤;外伤
blare[bleə(r)] *v*. 发出(响亮而刺耳的声音)

rib cage 肋架;胸廓

thrash [θræʃ] v. 激烈扭动,翻来覆去

choke [tʃəʊk] v. (使)窒息,哽噎

batter ['bætə(r)] v. 连续猛击;殴打

assemble [ə'sembl] v. 聚集;集合

neurosurgeon n. 神经外科医师

craniotomy [ˌkræni'ɒtəmi] n. 颅骨切开术

excruciating [ɪk'skruːʃieɪtɪŋ] adj. 极痛苦的

delirious [dɪ'lɪriəs] adj. 极度亢奋的,精神错乱的

writhe [raɪð] v. (常指因剧痛不停地)扭动,翻滚

the man's skull was so badly cracked that Apple could see his brain pulsing. She put both hands on his forehead, hoping to calm the **thrashing** victim. She gently pleaded with him to bear the pain just a little longer. "It's not your time to die!" she whispered. "You're still young."

In a **choked** whisper, he asked for her name.

"Dr. Sherry Apple," she replied.

"No. Your CB handle."

"How did you guess I have a CB?"

"Your voice ... I know your voice ..."

"My handle is Dr Froot Loops."

"Oh God ... It's me ... Woodpecker!"

Apple gasped—it was her truck driver. She leaned over the **battered** figure and said, "it's not your time, Woodpecker!"

The surgical team was **assembled**, and Key was rushed into the operating room. Apple and a **neurosurgeon** performed a **craniotomy**—a procedure to open the skull—to stop the bleeding and relieve pressure on the brain. The team labored nearly 24 hours.

The first days out of the operating room were **excruciating** for Woodpecker. He was **delirious**, and he **writhed** with fever. Often Apple would get home and find her phone ringing. Nurses, unable to calm

Woodpecker, asked her to return. She always did.

Gradually, after weeks of surgeries, his pain **ebbed**. About two months after his accident, he was ready to leave the hospital.

ebb[eb] v. 衰弱；衰退

As Woodpecker was pushed down the hallway in a wheelchair, he was **intercepted** by Apple, smiling.

intercept [ˌɪntəˈsept] v. 拦截；拦阻

"Well, look at you," she said.

She reached her hand out, and he took it in his. "I don't think I could have made it without you," he told her.

Apple's eyes welled up. "And I wouldn't have made it without you."

Task 1

1. Complete the following flow chart about Woody Key's experience in hospital.

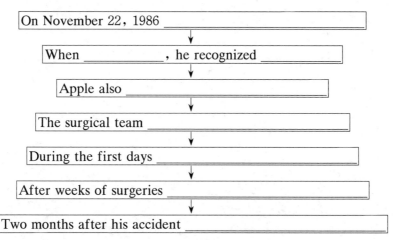

On November 22, 1986 _____

When _____, he recognized _____

Apple also _____

The surgical team _____

During the first days _____

After weeks of surgeries _____

Two months after his accident _____

2. Retell the process of Woody Key's treatment based on the chart. Connect the steps with appropriate connectives.

Task 2

In a TV interview program，Woody Key and Sherry Apple are invited to tell about their lifesaving coincidence. Narrate the story respectively as Woody Key and Sherry Apple.

Reading Aloud

A. 轻重规则(stressed and unstressed)

英语语句中的内容词(content words)又叫实意词,含有具体的语义内容,往往需要重读,包括名词、动词、形容词和副词。英语语句中的功能词(function words)仅体现语法功能关系,往往不需要重读,包括冠词、介词、连词、代词和助动词。简言之,重内容,轻功能。

如:Tom would accept his invitation.

They are building a greenhouse.

You know red is my favorite color.

Tell us about the exact story.

特殊情况:

1. 名词性的物主代词、指示代词、特殊疑问代词需要重读。

如:Ours are in the car. But theirs are missing.

That's for sure.

Why did you leave?

2. 当助动词与 not 缩写时,助动词需要重读。

如:They're coming to our party, aren't they?

I haven't been told about the accident.

B. Read aloud after the recording.

Dusk had descended quickly, and Sherry Apple knew she was in danger. Apple, a 34-year-old general-surgery intern, had been on call at Georgia Baptist Medical Center in Atlanta(now Atlanta Medical Center) for more than two days, with only a few hours' sleep. And now fatigue was clouding her eyes as she drove to a meeting in Louisville, Kentucky, nearly seven hours away.

She <u>tried</u> <u>snapping</u> on her <u>CB</u> <u>radio</u>，which <u>truckers</u> and <u>enthusiasts</u> <u>used</u> to <u>chat</u> and <u>warn</u> <u>one</u> <u>another</u> about <u>road</u> <u>conditions</u>，but the <u>airwaves</u> were <u>silent</u>. <u>Soon</u> the <u>hum</u> of the <u>tires</u> on the <u>blacktop</u> <u>became</u> an <u>eerie</u> <u>lullaby</u>，and <u>Apple</u> was <u>blinking</u> back <u>drowsiness</u>. Her <u>car</u> <u>started</u> to <u>weave</u>.

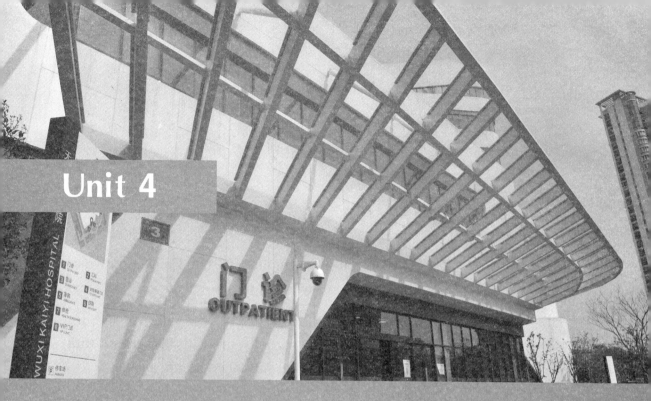

Unit 4

Upon completion of this unit，you will be able to：

- sort out sequence of a narration
- draw a mind map to clarify text's main ideas
- summarize the text in your own words
- identify key plots in a narration
- learn the pronunciation skill of reduction

✓音视频资源
✓参考答案
✓交流探讨

Text A

How Hubei Fought the Virus

[Doctors on the frontline in the Chinese province where the **coronavirus** outbroke tell Donna Lu about their experiences treating COVID-19.

WUHAN has partially lifted its **lockdown**, with the **epidemic** that spread through the city and out across the surrounding provinces of Hubei under control for the time being. In early April, *New Scientist* spoke to three doctors about life at the peak of the province's crisis.]

What were your roles in the coronavirus outbreak?

Xiang Lu: I led a medical aid team of more than 300 people from Jiangsu province to Huangshi [a city in Hubei province]. Our doctors were assigned to eight designated hospitals with coronavirus patients.

Zhiyong Peng: I manage the intensive care unit （ICU） at Zhongnan Hospital in Wuhan, with 30 doctors.

Yi Han: I first worked in the ICU at Wuhan First Hospital, and now I'm in Jinyintan Hospital. I'm currently looking after 13 critically ill patients, including four who are **intubated**, and one patient who

---

coronavirus [kəˈrəʊnəˈvaɪrəs] *n.* 冠状病毒

lockdown [ˈlɒkdaʊn] *n.* 活动（或行动）限制

epidemic [ˌepɪˈdemɪk] *n.* 流行病

intubate [ˈɪntjʊbeɪt] *v.* 把管子插进

is on **extracorporeal membrane oxygenation（ECMO）**.

When did you first arrive in Hubei province?

XL：Our team arrived in Huangshi on 11 February. The timeline in Huangshi was slightly behind that of Wuhan. The first patient admitted to the hospital［in Huangshi］was on 20 January. By the time we arrived，cases had **spiked** to around 700 patients in hospital and there were dozens of new patients being admitted every day. In total across Huangshi we had 100 critically ill patients.

YH：I arrived in Wuhan on 13 February. When we first came here，there were quite a lot of patients. At that time，we took over a ward with about 70 to 80 patients.

What was it like at the peak of the outbreak?

XL：At the peak，［Hubei province］had about 20,000 medical **personnel** from across China who came to help，working in more than 50 hospitals.

ZP：At the busiest，［the Zhongnan Hospital］had three ICU units looking after 44 critically ill COVID-19 patients. Our ICU is one of the biggest in Wuhan. From our experience，the average［ICU］**mortality** rate was around 25 to 30 per cent.

YH：At the busiest time，I was in the Wuhan First Hospital，working in the ECMO machine group. We worked for 6-hour shifts. The protective suit you wear is completely airtight，and the goggles and protective

extracorporeal membrane oxygenation （ECMO） ［ˌekstrəkɔːˈpɔːrɪəl ˈmembreɪn ˌɒksɪdʒəˈneɪʃn］体外膜肺氧合

spike［spaɪk］猛增；急升

personnel［ˌpɜːsəˈnel］n. (组织或军队中的)全体人员，职员

mortality［mɔːˈtælətɪ］n. 死亡数量；死亡率；死亡

dehydration
[ˌdiːhaɪˈdreɪʃən] *n*. 脱水

mask make your whole body tired. After 6 hours，you feel like collapsing. Every time you come out，the overwhelming feeling is："I have to drink a mouthful of water，otherwise I might die of **dehydration**." I had no concept of time at all，just working and trying to rest as much as possible during the short downtime.

Were there any shortages?

YH：At the busiest time，there weren't enough supplies. There were bed shortages，too. We didn't have enough equipment until the middle of February. From a national level，we were then supplied with a lot of high-end machines，including **ventilators** and ECMO machines. Now there's not really any equipment issues. But even now，we are trying not to be wasteful.

ventilator [ˈventɪleɪtə(r)] *n*. 通气机；呼吸器

XL：At the most stressful time，we didn't have enough beds or ventilators. There wasn't even enough oxygen. The Huangshi infectious diseases hospital used to be for patients with mild disease，but suddenly it was treating so many severe and critically ill cases. We needed to use five to eight ventilators in a ward at once，but the oxygen pressure wasn't high enough. We then started transferring severely ill patients to the Huangshi Central Hospital，which had a better-equipped ICU.

How are things now?

YH：The overall situation is better. There are still a small number of [COVID-19] patients in Jinyintan Hospital receiving treatment. From the perspective of medical staff, even if there's a rise in cases again, we are now experienced in dealing with this problem.

ZP: We have almost no new cases in our hospital now. All the COVID-19 patients will be transferred to a new hospital, Huoshenshan, in about a week's time. There are about 200 or 300 patients in total still in hospital in Wuhan.

XL: In total, Huangshi had 1,015 patients and 39 deaths. About 2,800 healthcare workers from Jiangsu province went to Hubei, and now most of them have returned and are **quarantining**. After our team [of 300] came back to quarantine, our tests have all come back negative and nobody has been infected.

quarantine ['kwɒrəntiːn] v. /n. (对动物或人)进行检疫,隔离

What has working away from home been like?

ZP: We have to [stay] in a hotel and can't go home, for more than two months already. We work for three weeks and then have one week off. The hospital authorities have invited psychologists to come to our department to talk with our personnel in ICU, and also provide support for living and eating.

XL: Our team lived in three hotels. You had to use the **shuttle bus** to commute to work. We ate while quarantined too, in our rooms without **congregating** in a dining hall. Everyone was maintaining social distancing.

shuttle bus ['ʃʌtl bʌs] 区间(公共汽)车

congregate ['kɒŋgrɪgeɪt] v. 群集;聚集;集合

YH: Our Jiangsu team is still here in Wuhan. We might be the last to leave. We might go home in mid-

April，but we haven't been given the directive yet. I haven't seen my child for a long time.

What measures worked well while treating patients?

ZP：All medical staff received regular testing，every three to four weeks. There was additional testing if you had symptoms or if one of your colleagues was infected. It was very important to protect all our medical staff.

XL：In terms of managing patients with COVID-19，I personally think that preventing mild cases worsening to severe or even critical illness is important，by intervening early. The approach we take is the same as for other **inflammatory** responses. If a patient's level of ［the signalling molecule］ **interleukin**-6 is high，we use **monoclonal antibodies** to suppress the generation of a **cytokine storm** ［a severe and acute inflammatory response］. But this needs to be done early. If the patient's situation is already very serious，then often it's too late and nothing you do will work.

YH：I think China's most effective approach to fighting this epidemic is that it has the space to quarantine these patients. The vast majority of patients with mild cases can effectively recover without transmitting the virus to others，so long as you give them the space to quarantine，with medical support and treatment as needed.

inflammatory [ɪnˈflæmətrɪ] *adj.* 发炎的

interleukin [ˌɪntəˈluːkɪn] n. 白细胞介素

monoclonal [ˌmɒnəˈkloʊnəl] *adj.* 单细胞系的；单克隆的

antibody [ˈæntɪbɒdɪ] *n.* 抗体

cytokine storm [ˈsaɪtoʊkiːn stɔːm] 细胞因子风暴；细胞因子暴

Do you have any advice for other countries?

YH：One point—the most basic and，I think，the most difficult—is that you must provide ample space and facilities for people to quarantine. Having adequate facilities to screen patients is also important，including temperature testing and **nucleic acid** and antibody testing kits.

nucleic acid ［njuːˌkliːɪk ˈæsɪd］ *n.* 核酸

Personal protective equipment is also important. My patients who are being treated are asked to wear masks when they can—even if they are on supplementary oxygen.

Worry is **warranted** but it's not necessary to panic. We should pay attention to social distancing and self-isolation. Protective materials such as masks should be worn if you are feeling unwell，even if you just have a cold.

warrant ［ˈwɒrənt］ *v.* 使有必要；使正当；使恰当

Task 1

Put the following occurrences in order of time.

_____The coronavirus broke out in Hubei.

_____The epidemic that spread through the city and out across the surrounding provinces of Hubei was under control.

_____Wuhan partially lifted its lockdown.

_____Dr Xiang Lu led a medical aid team of more than 300 people from Jiangsu province to Huangshi.

_____In Huangshi，the first COVID-19 patient was admitted to the hospital on 20 January.

_____All the COVID-19 patients in Wuhan were transferred to a new hospital，Huoshenshan.

_____Cases reached around 700 patients in hospital in Huangshi and there were dozens of new patients being admitted every day.

_____Dr Yi Han's team arrived in Wuhan.

Task 2

Draw a mind map to illustrate "How Hubei fought the virus" based on what you learn from the text.

Task 3

Introduce "How Hubei fought the virus" to others with the help of the mind map in Task 2.

Text B

A Shift with Medic 61

By Charlotte Alter / Yonkers, N. Y.

Alanna Badgley wakes up with a sense of doom. Her alarm goes off at 4:45 a. m., but she lies there breathing until 5:15: in through her nose, and out through her mouth. Then she throws off the covers, splashes some water on her face, brushes her teeth and puts on her uniform.

The Westchester County, New York, **paramedic** normally has an Eggo waffle with peanut butter and Nutella for breakfast, but lately she's too nervous to eat. Her boyfriend, Rudy Green, has packed her a jar of cut fruit and a Ziploc baggie of veggies, which is pretty much all she can stomach these days. Badgley stuffs it into her JanSport backpack and walks to the Empress Emergency Medical Services base in Yonkers, N. Y., clocking in just before 6 a.m. on April 1.

She checks her gear: **intubation** kits, an oxygen pressure mask, an alternative airway device. She's been wearing the same N95 mask for two weeks. Someone **squawks** over the loudspeaker, calling for Medic 61. "That's me," she says.

medic ['medɪk] *n.* 医师；卫生员

paramedic [ˌpærəˈmedɪk] *n.* 护理人员；医务辅助人员

intubation [ˌɪntjuˈbeɪʃən] *n.* 插管；插管法

squawk [skwɔːk] *v.* 发出刺耳的尖叫声；尖声高叫

hoarder [ˈhɔːdə(r)] *n.* 囤积者，囤积狂

bedbug [ˈbedbʌg] *n.* 臭虫；床虱

infest [ɪnˈfest] *v.* 大量滋生

pandemic [pænˈdemɪk] *n.* （全国或全球性）流行病；大流行病

Badgley，28，is small and sharp，with the quick，sure movements of a paramedic who knows exactly what she's doing. She responds to 911 calls with emergency medical technicians（EMTs）but typically gets the cases that require advanced medical help. Lately，that means patients with COVID-19. She can do much of what ER doctors do，often in less optimal conditions. She's dug through **hoarders'** homes to reach her patients，responded to car accidents and sudden births，and once intubated a man while lying on her belly on his **bedbug-infested** carpet.

Paramedics like Badgley are now the first line of defense in a global **pandemic**，and Westchester County has been one of the nation's hardest hit. But with doctors overwhelmed and hospitals forbidding visitors，paramedics like Badgley are also taking on an additional role：they are often the first medical professional seen by patients in distress and the last one seen in person by their families.

It's often up to Badgley to tell patients' families that they can't ride in the ambulance and can't come to the hospital. She stands there as they slowly realize that her arrival could mean a permanent good-bye. Badgley tries to make up for it in the ambulance. She holds patients' hands，rubs their backs and provides the one-on-one comfort she knows they're unlikely to get at crowded hospitals. "I'm there to talk to them," she says，"and to provide some level of empathy and humanity in the moment in which they are truly terrified. "

The first call of the day comes in at 6:58 a.m.: a car accident on the Sprain Brook Parkway. At 7:28, the radio squawks again. This time the **dispatcher** says, " Screening positive ": the patient is exhibiting symptoms of COVID-19. As Badgley puts on her **siren**, she hears a second, separate call coming in for " 30 Alpha 2 "—Green's **identifier**. She smiles when she hears it: the paramedic version of running into your boyfriend at the office.

Badgley and Green met on the job three years ago. For the past three weeks, they've spent most of their working hours responding to 911 calls about COVID-19. Nine co-workers have tested positive, she says. Many others have called out sick but haven't been officially diagnosed. At this point, Badgley and Green figure they both have the virus already, and if they don't, they will soon. "We had a conversation about 'How would you want to be buried? Do you want to be **cremated**?'" she recalls. She told Green she'd like to be buried under a tree in a **biodegradable** bag.

At 7:41, Badgley arrives at a brick apartment building across from a boarded-up church in north Yonkers. She puts on goggles and her N95 mask, hooks her surgical mask over her ears, grabs her big blue bag and heads inside. The patient is a woman in her 70s who speaks only Spanish. She has severe **abdominal** pain, a high fever and low oxygen levels. As

dispatcher [dɪˈspætʃə(r)]
n. 调度员
siren [ˈsaɪrən] n. 汽笛;警报器

identifier [aɪˈdentɪfaɪə(r)]
n. 标识符,标识号

cremate [krəˈmeɪt] v. 焚烧,火化(尸体)
biodegradable
[ˌbaɪəʊdɪˈgreɪdəbl] adj.
可生物降解的

abdominal [æbˈdɒmɪnl]
adj. 腹部的

stretcher ['stretʃə(r)] *n*. 担架

footage ['fʊtɪdʒ] *n*. （影片中的）连续镜头，片段

the EMTs get her onto the **stretcher**, Badgley sees the Spanish-language news channel airing **footage** of paramedics responding to COVID patients.

An hour later, there's another squawk over the radio: a patient at a nursing home. "Screening positive." It's a woman in a green top, moaning and nearly unconscious, her lips and fingers blue. "Can you tell me your name?" Badgley asks. "Can you tell me where you are?" The only sound from the woman is a groan. She needs to be intubated, but it won't be easy to do here. An intubation is an **aerosolizing** procedure, which means it sprays tiny **virus-laden** particles into the air. You'd want to wear a Tyvek suit and face shield for a procedure like that.

aerosolize [eərə'səʊlaɪs] *v*. 使成烟雾状散开，雾化

virus-laden 带病毒的

Instead, Badgley gives the patient nasal oxygen as she wheels her to the ambulance and then an oxygen mask once they get inside. As her oxygen levels rise, the woman improves enough to mumble her name. "Hold my hand, hold my hand, hold my hand," Badgley says. "It's OK."

At 10:05, another radio call: "Patient screening positive." When Badgley arrives at the cream-and-yellow house, there's a tree blossoming outside. The patient has a fever, shortness of breath and chest pain. "Straight-up COVID," Badgley says. He's conscious, and strong enough to walk slowly to the ambulance with a pulse **oximeter** attached to his finger to see if his oxygen level drops as he walks. (It does.) His cough

oximeter ['ɒksɪmiːtə] *n*. 血氧计；血氧仪

sounds like a barking seal.

Radio call at 10:57: "Screening inconclusive." It's an older man who fell and injured his arm after feeling weak and dizzy. "But why was he weak?" Badgley asks rhetorically. Probably COVID. At 11:58: "Screening positive," an unresponsive patient in Mount Vernon.

By the end of her shift at 6 p.m., Badgley will have taken 11 calls, nine of them for suspected coronavirus patients. The patients are middle-aged and old, black and white, living in places from Victorian houses to nursing homes. Most have fever and shortness of breath, but the symptoms can vary. Badgley has noticed only one common thread: "The identifying feature is fear."

EMTs and paramedics are trained to respond fearlessly to scenes of sudden catastrophe. They're prepared for emergencies, but emergencies don't usually last this long. It's **upended** Badgley's sense of space and time. "In some ways you're looking into the future," Badgley explains. In the scenes of devastation in Italy and China, "you can see where we're headed," she says. "But in some ways, because of the lag of the data in the testing, you're also looking into the past."

upend [ʌpˈend] v. 翻倒；使颠倒

The patients she treats today were likely infected a week ago. Next week she'll respond to calls for patients infected today. Fighting COVID is like racing toward a star that may have burned out centuries ago but whose light is only just now reaching the eye.

reception [rɪ'sepʃn] *n.*
接待处；接待区
gurney ['gɜːnɪ] *n.*（医院
中推送病人用的）轮床
maneuver [mə'nuːvə] *v.*
（使某物）移动，运动；熟练
而巧妙地引导
orderly ['ɔːdəlɪ] *n.*（医院
的）护工，勤杂工

wind [waɪnd] *v.* 使喘不
过气来；使喘大气

When she needs to take a bathroom break, Badgley goes into St. Joseph's Medical Center in Yonkers. The **reception** area is crowded with **gurneys**, and she has to **maneuver** around people lying on beds in the halls. On her way to the restroom, she runs into a friend, an **orderly** who is tasked with putting the dead into body bags. They had both been planning vacations in Jamaica. Instead, they are doing this.

Another call comes through at 2:42 p.m., for a man with difficulty breathing: "Screening positive." Badgley hangs her head, takes a deep breath and turns on her siren. At 2:46, she arrives at a brick apartment building. The patient is a 45-year-old man with a high fever and chest pain. He can't walk from one room to another without getting **winded**. He has no appetite and can't keep food down. He tested positive for COVID, he says. His wife has symptoms too.

"I know you're in a lot of pain, OK? But the most important thing is just to try to focus on breathing," Badgley tells him. "Slowly in through your nose, slowly out through your mouth, OK?"

While the EMTs get the man onto the stretcher, his wife pulls Badgley aside. "Please, I want him to be OK," she says. He has already been to St. Joseph's and doesn't want to be sent back. They want him to go to a hospital in the Bronx. But Badgley's team is only authorized to take him to an in-county hospital.

"Please don't let him die," the woman says.

"We won't let him die in our ambulance," Badgley says. Can she guarantee that? Of course she can't.

This is the worst part. Before coronavirus, she could take a family member in the ambulance or tell them to meet the patient at the hospital. She'd know that the family would get to sit by the bedside and direct their questions to the doctor. Now she's not only treating the patient but managing a goodbye.

The woman is crying as the EMTs are wheeling her husband away. "I'll pray for you," Badgley says. "You pray for you. And breathe." Normally, she would hug the woman, but hugs aren't allowed anymore. Instead, Badgley grips both of the woman's hands in her gloved fingers. The woman is melting in panic. Badgley knows she is realizing this may be the last time she sees her husband.

"You breathe, he breathes, everybody focuses on breathing, OK?" Badgley says. The woman tries. "There you go. Exactly," Badgley says. "This is the most important time to focus on breathing. OK? All right. That's the first thing. Breathing."

Breathing, Badgley thinks, is the beginning of it all. The very first thing any of us ever did in our life was breathe. The woman calms down as she takes in air. The patient is already downstairs at the ambulance with the EMTs. Badgley grabs her bag and heads to the elevator. The doors close, and Badgley stands there in silence, wearing her two-week-old mask after her ninth coronavirus patient of the day. She has two hours left on her shift. Tomorrow she will come back to work and put on the same mask. She will lose two patients that shift，dead before they even make it to the ambulance. But she doesn't know that yet. For now，she's just focused on breathing：in through her nose，and out through her mouth.

Task 1

How does Alanna Badgley spend this day—April 1，2020? Fill out the chart according to the time.

Time of the day	What Alanna Badgley does
4:45 a.m.	Badgley's alarm clock sounds.
5:15 a.m.	
Just before 6 a.m.	
6:58 a.m.	
7:28 a.m.	
7:41 a.m.	Badgley arrives at _____ and begins tending and escorting a lady in her 70s.
An hour later	She receives another call and begins _____ _____.
10:05 a.m.	
10:57 a.m.	
11:58 a.m.	She receives another call to aid _____.
2:42 p.m.	
2:46 p.m.	Badgley arrives at the patient's apartment. Apart from tending the man，she also _____.
The rest of her shift before 6 p.m.	Badgley receives 4 more emergency calls and keeps on working without rest.

Task 2

Come up with questions about the text. The questions can be about the main idea or important details of the story. They can also be inference drawn from the text or lessons learned.

Model question:

1. Why does Alanna Badgley have a sense of doom when she wakes up?

2. _____

3. _____

4. _____

5. _____

6. _____

Task 3

Answer the questions in Task 2.

Model question & answer:

1. Why does Alanna Badgley have a sense of doom when she wakes up?

"A sense of doom" depicts Badgley's desperate emotion. As a paramedic, she has to take on her responsibility to help with the emergent cases. However confronted with highly contagious dreadful coronavirus and inadequate medical staff and equipment, she feels weak and helpless.

2. _____

_____

_____

_____

_____

3. _____

_____

_____

_____

_____

4. _____

_____

_____

_____

5. _____

_____

_____

_____

6. _____

_____

_____

_____

Reading Aloud

A. 弱化现象(reduction)1

英语中的功能词在轻读的基础上往往还需要进一步弱化,它们通常有强式和弱式两种读法,如介词 at 的强式为/æt/,弱式为/ət/。功能词出现在语句末尾时,一般轻读;在句首时,可以轻读也可以弱化,弱化更多出现在快速话语中。

常见弱化规律:

1. 紧张的元音弱化成放松的元音。

2. 其他元音都弱化为中元音/ə/。

3. 省略常用功能词中的元音或辅音,如 and 缩略成 n。

常见功能词的弱化:

1. 冠词——a/ə/、an/ən/, the/ðə /(辅音前)或/ðɪ/(在元音前)

<u>a</u> dog   <u>an</u> applc   <u>the</u> country   <u>the</u> orange

2. 介词——to/tə/, for/fə/, from/frəm/, at/ət/, of/əv/或/ə/

go <u>to</u> school look <u>for</u> me   come <u>from</u> China

look <u>at</u> the book   full <u>of</u> water   a lot <u>of</u> people

3. 连词——and/ənd/,/ən/或/n/, but/bət/, or/ə/, as/əz/, than/ðən/, because /bɪkəz/或/kəz/, who/hʊ/和 whose/hʊz/

I had bread <u>and</u> butter <u>for</u> breakfast.

He came <u>in and</u> turned <u>on</u> the light.

4. 人称代词——me/mɪ/,we/wɪ/, us/əs/或/s/, you/jə/(在辅音前)或/jʊ/(在元音前), your/jə/, he/hɪ/或/ɪ/, him/ɪm/, his/ɪz/, she/ʃɪ/, her/hə/或/ə/, them/ðəm/或/əm/, their/ðə/

I want <u>you</u> to help <u>them</u>.

Tell <u>her</u> <u>she</u> is <u>their</u> best friend.

B. Read aloud after the recording.

1. In early April, *New Scientist* spoke to three doctors about life at the peak of the province's crisis.

2. I led a medical aid team of more than 300 people from Jiangsu province to Huangshi, a city in Hubei province.

3. I have to drink a mouthful of water, otherwise I might die of dehydration.

4. We needed to use five to eight ventilators in a ward at once, but the oxygen pressure wasn't high enough.

5. The hospital authorities have invited psychologists to come to our department to talk with our personnel in ICU, and also provide support for living and eating.

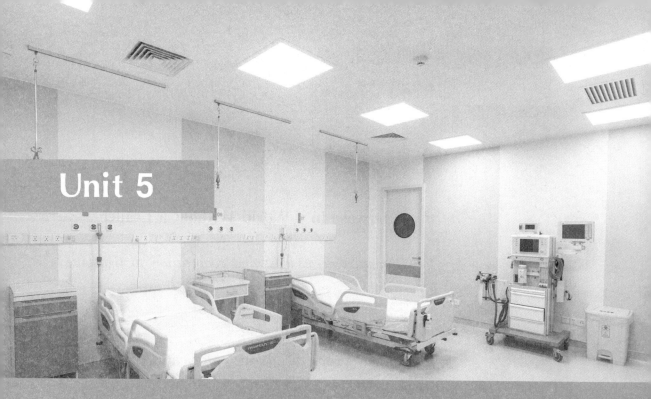

Unit 5

Upon completion of this unit，you will be able to：

- identify figures of speech and paraphrase the sentences
- deliver a presentation about the text
- summarize diagnostic and therapeutic procedure
- learn the pronunciation skill of reduction

✓音视频资源
✓参考答案
✓交流探讨

Text A

Disease in a World Without a Leader

—Humanity needs trust and cooperation to fight the pandemic

By Yuval Noah Harari

Many people blame the coronavirus epidemic on **globalization** and say the only way to prevent more such outbreaks is to **deglobalize** the world：build walls，restrict travel，reduce trade. However，while short-term quarantine is essential to stop epidemics，long-term **isolationism** will lead to economic collapse without offering any real protection against **infectious** diseases. Just the opposite. The real anti-dote to epidemics is cooperation.

Epidemics killed millions of people long before the current age of globalization. In the 14th century，there were no airplanes or **cruise ships**，and yet the Black Death spread from East Asia to Western Europe in little more than a decade，killing at least a quarter of the population. In 1520，Mexico had no trains or even donkeys，yet it took only a year for a **smallpox** epidemic to **decimate** up to a third of its inhabitants. In 1918，a particularly **virulent strain** of flu managed to

---

globalization [ˌɡləʊbəlaɪˈzeɪʃn] *n.* 全球化

deglobalize [diːˈɡləʊbəlaɪz] *v.* 去全球化

isolationism [ˌaɪsəˈleɪʃənɪzəm] *n.* 孤立主义

infectious [ɪnˈfekʃəs] *adj.* 传染性的

cruise ship [kruːz ʃɪp] *n.* 大型游轮

smallpox [ˈsmɔːlpɒks] *n.* 天花

decimate [ˈdesɪmeɪt] *v.* 大量毁灭，大批杀死（某地区的动物、植物或人）

virulent [ˈvɪrələnt] *adj.* 致命的；剧毒的

strain [streɪn] *n.* 品种；（疾病的）类型

spread within a few months to the remotest corners of the world. It infected more than a quarter of the human species and killed tens of millions.

In the century that passed since 1918, humankind has become ever more vulnerable to epidemics, because of a combination of growing populations and better transport. Today a virus can travel business class across the world in 24 hours and infect **megacities** of millions. We should therefore have expected to live in an infectious hell, with one deadly plague after another.

megacity ['megəˌsɪtɪ] n. 特大都市,大城市

However, both the incidence and impact of epidemics have actually gone down dramatically. Despite **horrendous** outbreaks such as AIDS and **Ebola**, epidemics kill a far smaller proportion of humans in the 21st century than in any previous time since the Stone Age. This is because the best defense humans have against **pathogens** is not isolation; it is information. Humanity has been winning the war against epidemics because in the arms race between pathogens and doctors, pathogens rely on blind **mutations** while doctors rely on the scientific analysis of information.

horrendous [həˈrendəs] adj. 令人震惊的;可怕的

Ebola [ɪˈbəʊlə] n. 埃博拉

pathogen [ˈpæθədʒən] n. 病原体

mutation [mjuːˈteɪʃn] n. (生物物种的)变异,突变

During the past century, scientists, doctors and nurses throughout the world have pooled information and together managed to understand both the **mechanism** behind epidemics and the means of countering them. The theory of evolution explained

mechanism [ˈmekənɪzəm] n. 机制

erupt [ɪˈrʌpt] v. 突然发生；爆发

vaccination [ˌvæksɪˈneɪʃən] n. 接种疫苗；种痘
antibiotic [ˌæntɪbaɪˈɒtɪk] n. 抗生素
hygiene [ˈhaɪdʒiːn] n. 卫生
infrastructure [ˈɪnfrəstrʌktʃə(r)] n. 基础设施
predator [ˈpredətə (r)] n. 捕食性动物；掠夺者
medieval [ˌmediˈiːvl] adj. 中世纪的

solidarity [ˌsɒlɪˈdærəti] n. 团结；齐心协力

catastrophe [kəˈtæstrəfi] n. 灾难；灾祸
ostracize [ˈɒstrəsaɪz] v. 排挤；排斥

why and how new diseases **erupt** and old diseases become more virulent. Genetics enabled scientists to spy on the pathogens' own instruction manual. Once scientists understood what causes epidemics, it became much easier to fight them. **Vaccinations**, **antibiotics**, improved **hygiene** and a much better medical **infrastructure** have allowed humanity to gain the upper hand over its invisible **predators**.

What does this history teach us for the current coronavirus epidemic? First, it implies that you cannot protect yourself by permanently closing your borders. Remember that epidemics spread rapidly even in the Middle Ages, long before the age of globalization. So even if you reduce your global connections to the level of a **medieval** kingdom, that still would not be enough. To really protect yourself through isolation, you would have to go back to the Stone Age. Can you do that?

Second, history indicates that real protection comes from the sharing of reliable scientific information, and from global **solidarity**. When one country is struck by an epidemic, it should be willing to honestly share information about the outbreak without fear of economic **catastrophe**—while other nations should be able to trust that information, and should be willing to extend a helping hand rather than **ostracize** the victim.

International cooperation is needed also for effective quarantine measures. Quarantine and lockdown are essential for stopping the spread of epidemics. But when countries distrust one another and each country feels that it is on its own, governments hesitate to take such drastic measures. If you discover 100 coronavirus cases in your country, would you immediately lock down entire cities and regions? To a large extent, that depends on what you expect from other countries. Locking down your own cities could lead to economic collapse. If you think other countries will then come to your aid, you will be more likely to adopt this drastic measure sooner.

Perhaps the most important thing people should realize about such epidemics is that the spread of an epidemic in any country endangers the entire human species. In the 1970s, humanity managed to completely **eradicate** the smallpox virus because all people in all nations were **vaccinated** against smallpox. If even one country failed to vaccinate its population, it could have endangered the whole of humankind, because as long as the smallpox virus existed and evolved somewhere, it could always spread again everywhere.

eradicate [ɪˈrædɪkeɪt] v. 根除；消灭；杜绝

vaccinate [ˈvæksɪneɪt] v. 给……接种疫苗

In the fight against viruses, humanity needs to closely guard borders. But not the borders between countries. Rather, it needs to guard the border between the human world and the virus-sphere. Planet Earth is **teeming with** countless viruses, and new viruses are constantly evolving because of genetic mutations. The borderline separating this virus-sphere from the

teem with [tiːm wɪð] 充满

human world passes inside the body of each and every human being. If a dangerous virus manages to penetrate this border anywhere on earth, it puts the whole human species in danger.

Over the past century, humanity has fortified this border like never before. Modern health care systems have been built to serve as a wall on that border, and nurses, doctors and scientists are the guards who patrol it and repel intruders. However, long sections of this border have been left **woefully** exposed. There are hundreds of millions of people around the world who lack even basic health care services. This endangers all of us. We are used to thinking about health in national terms, but providing better health care for Iranians helps protect Israelis and Americans too from epidemics. This simple truth should be obvious to everyone.

Today, humanity faces an acute crisis not only because of the coronavirus, but also because of the lack of trust between humans. To defeat an epidemic, people need to trust scientific experts, citizens need to trust public authorities, and countries need to trust one another. Over the past few years, irresponsible politicians have deliberately undermined trust in science, in public authorities and in international cooperation. As a result, we are now facing this crisis **bereft of** global leaders who can inspire, organize and finance a coordinated global response.

woefully ['wəʊf(ə)lɪ] *adv*. 悲伤地；不幸地

bereft of [bɪ'reftəv] 失去；丧失

During the 2014 Ebola epidemic, the US served as that kind of leader. The US fulfilled a similar role also during the 2008 financial crisis, when it **rallied** behind enough countries to prevent a global economic **meltdown**. But in recent years the US has resigned its role as a global leader. The current US. Administration has cut support for international organizations and has made it very clear to the world that the US no longer has any real friends, only interests.

rally ['rælɪ] v. 召集；集合

meltdown ['meltdaʊn] n. 崩溃，彻底失败

The **void** left by the US has not been filled by anyone else. **Xenophobia**, isolationism and distrust now characterize most of the international system. Without trust and global solidarity, we will not be able to stop the coronavirus epidemic.

void [vɔɪd] n. 空间；空白

xenophobia [ˌzenəˈfəʊbɪə] n. 仇外，惧外（对外国人的厌恶或惧怕）

If this epidemic results in greater disunity and mistrust among humans, it will be the virus' greatest victory. When humans **squabble**, viruses double. In contrast, if the epidemic results in closer global cooperation, it will be a victory not only against the coronavirus, but against all future pathogens.

squabble ['skwɒbl] v. （为琐事）争吵，发生口角

Task 1

What are the figures of speech in the following sentences? Rephrase the sentences in your own words.

1. We should therefore have expected to live in an infectious hell, with one deadly plague after another.

2. Humanity has been winning the war against epidemics because in the arms race between pathogens and doctors, pathogens rely on blind mutations while doctors rely on the scientific analysis of information.

3. Vaccinations, antibiotics, improved hygiene and a much better medical infrastructure have allowed humanity to gain the upper hand over its invisible predators.

4. Modern health care systems have been built to serve as a wall on that border, and nurses, doctors and scientists are the guards who patrol it and repel intruders.

5. However, long sections of this border have been left woefully exposed.

6. When humans squabble, viruses double.

Task 2

Based on the text, deliver a presentation about how to fight the pandemic. Prepare PPT and write a transcript.

Sample PPT slide:

How to fight the pandemic

Overview

- Globalization is not to blame
- What does history teach us
- What kind of world we are facing
- Conclusion

Globalization is not to blame

- Epidemics before globalization _____
  1. In the 14th century, Black Death _____

  _____

  2. _____
  3. _____
- During the past century _____

What does history teach us

- First, _____
- Second, _____

What kind of world we are facing

- _____
- _____

Conclusion

- disunity and mistrust→ _____
- _____ → _____

Transcript

As the article suggests, confronted with coronavirus pandemic, some blame globalization as the bad guy. Starting with defying this charge, the author points out the real anti-dote to the pandemic by looking back into the history and analyzing today's world.

In order to prove that globalization is not to blame, _____

_____

_____

Moving on to the second part, the article points out that, to combat today's enemy, we must learn from history. _____

_____

_____

_____

However, the author is deeply disturbed by the current situation. _____

_____

_____

_____

Finally, alarm is sounded. _____

_____

_____

Text B

Growing Pains

〔Doctors find a surprising cause for a preteen's stomach pain and high blood pressure.〕

By Amitha Kalaichandran

Life was changing fast for Ameera. She had moved with her family thousands of miles from the Middle East to Canada, and had just started school as a sixth-grader.

The 11-year-old was excited but also anxious, and she started to complain of stomach pain. Eventually her parents took her to their family doctor.

During the exam, the doctor discovered that Ameera's blood pressure was higher than it should have been for her age. So, she ordered an **ultrasound** of her **kidneys**, since they help **regulate** blood pressure. The test revealed she had a mass near her right kidney, and she was referred to the local children's hospital, where I and other doctors examined her.

Ameera spoke in a quiet voice. She answered most questions by nodding yes or no, as her parents sat nearby. They said that over the last few weeks, Ameera felt **nauseous**, had to **urinate** often and was

ultrasound 〔ˈʌltrəsaʊnd〕 n. 超声波扫描检查
kidney 〔ˈkɪdnɪ〕 n. 肾;肾脏
regulate 〔ˈreɡjuleɪt〕 v. 约束,控制

nauseous 〔ˈnɔːzɪəs〕 adj. 恶心的;想呕吐的
urinate 〔ˈjʊərɪneɪt〕 v. 排尿;小便

often thirsty. The skin around her eyes was puffy. And Ameera's blood pressure was indeed high，measuring 140/90 (A healthy range for her age and height is between 90/60 and 120/80).

abdomen ['æbdəmən] *n.* 腹(部)

hip [hɪp] *n.* 臀部；髋

As she lay on her back on the exam table，I felt her **abdomen** and located a mass just above her right **hip**，toward her back. She winced when I pressed it softly. I had her sit up，then examined her kidneys by pressing at the midback，just above the hips. Everything there seemed normal.

nephrotic syndrome 肾病综合征

fluid ['fluːɪd] *n.* 液体

However，her urine test showed high protein levels，which suggested **nephrotic syndrome**，a kidney disorder. The disorder can also cause **fluid** to build up around the eyes and ankles，as well as high blood pressure. It explained nearly all her symptoms，but not the mass and the pain.

ovary ['əʊvərɪ] *n.* 卵巢

bladder ['blædə(r)] *n.* 膀胱

Surgery was the only way to get a good look at the mass. We didn't know if it was affecting her **ovaries** or **bladder**，so we needed a variety of specialists at the operation.

Something Amiss

After starting the procedure，we were shocked to find that Ameera's mass—large for her body，about the size of a plum—seemed to grow out of her right ovary.

Then another shock：Ameera had no left ovary. Instead，she had an underdeveloped ovary—merely tissue—known as a **streak**. She also had no **uterus**.

That combination of missing organs is rare，and it had implications beyond Ameera not being able to bear children：Something may have gone **awry** in her body's development at the **embryo** stage. Now came the hard work of figuring out exactly what was ahead of us.

We took tissue sample of the kidneys and the mass. Ameera did indeed have a kidney disease，explaining her nephrotic syndrome symptoms. And the mass was a **gonadoblastoma**，a type of tumor that was not **cancerous**，but could eventually become so. We made plans to remove it in a subsequent surgery.

Such tumors are found in a few known diseases，such as **Swyer syndrome**，in which patients have neither ovaries nor **testes**，or Denys-Drash syndrome，which usually includes a specific type of kidney tumor called a **Wilms tumor**. She had neither of these. One other syndrome seemed quite possible，but determining whether she had it meant learning a bit more about Ameera.

So，after her surgery，we drew blood for further testing. All we could do now was wait，and hope this would finally reveal what caused her illness.

Finally，an Explanation

After an anxious week，we finally received the test results：an XY **genotype**. According to her **chromosomes**，Ameera was male.

---

tissue ['tɪʃuː] n.（人、动植物细胞的）组织

streak [striːk] n. 条纹；条痕

uterus ['juːtərəs] n. 子宫

awry [ə'raɪ] adv. / adj. 出错；出岔子；歪；斜

embryo ['embriəʊ] n. 胚；胚胎

gonadoblastoma [gəʊneɪdəʊ'blæstəʊmə] n. 性腺胚细胞瘤

cancerous ['kænsərəs] adj. 癌的；癌性的

Swyer syndrome ['swaɪə 'sɪndrəʊm] 性腺发育不全；斯威尔症候群

testis ['testiːz] n. 睾丸

Wilms tumor 肾母细胞瘤；威尔姆氏肿瘤

genotype ['dʒenətaɪp] n. 基因型

chromosome ['krəʊməsəʊm] n. 染色体

Most humans have 23 sets of chromosomes, which contain genes that dictate how we develop, our appearance and many other features. One set of chromosomes determines biologic sex: XX for female or XY for male. All human embryos effectively begin as females, the default pathway for development. But early on, the presence of a Y chromosome halts formation of female **reproductive** organs such as the ovaries and uterus. These embryos usually develop testes and male **genitalia** instead—unless something occurs to stop it.

reproductive [ˌriːprəˈdʌktɪv] *adj.* 生殖的；繁殖的
genitalia [dʒɛnəˈtɑːljə] *n.* 外生殖器；外阴部

Having an XY genotype explained why Ameera's left ovary was barely formed. It also explained why she had no uterus. And yet, her body did not produce enough male **hormone** to allow for formation of a male reproductive system.

hormone [ˈhɔːməʊn] *n.* 激素；荷尔蒙

It's unclear what caused this **disruption**, but it led Ameera to be chromosomally male, despite her **external** female genitalia.

disruption [dɪsˈrʌpʃn] *n.* 中断；扰乱；混乱
external [ɪkˈstɜːnl] *adj.* 外部的

We could now finally explain Ameera's symptoms with a single diagnosis. With the XY genotype, nephrotic syndrome and gonadoblastoma, Ameera showed the classic signs of Frasier syndrome. It's a rare condition that affects about 1 in 100,000 live births.

In most cases, the syndrome shows up as an XY male with slightly unusual male genitalia who complains of kidney symptoms.

In girls who haven't yet had their periods, like Ameera, the only hint of Frasier syndrome might be high blood pressure. If it's not caught early, the condition could lead to kidney failure and **transformation** of the tumor to a cancer.

We removed the mass surgically, and her right ovary—which turned out to be a partially formed testis—eventually had to come out too, due to the risk of its cells turning cancerous.

Treatment of the nephrotic syndrome (namely through blood pressure measurement and water pills) and surgery were essential components of her recovery, which went well.

A Support System

After the operation, we had a longer discussion with Ameera's family. At first, they didn't understand the diagnosis, and since she had been raised female, they were unclear as to how that might change as she matured. It was extra complicated because Ameera **hailed from** a traditional and conservative Middle Eastern family, where gender roles are strictly defined.

That said, her family was ready to help Ameera through the process, whatever that might **entail**. Her Frasier syndrome didn't necessarily mean Ameera would identify as male, female or other, since gender is self-identified and doesn't always correlate with biologic sex. It also didn't necessarily **confer** a specific

---

transformation [ˌtrænsfəˈmeɪʃn] *n.* 变化,转变

hail from [heɪl frəm]出身于;来自

entail [ɪnˈteɪl] *v.* 牵涉;需要;使必要

confer [kənˈfɜː(r)] *v.* 赋予,授予

sexual orientation
[ˈsekʃuəl ˌɔːrɪənˈteɪʃn] 性
取向

sexual orientation.

At our suggestion，her family enrolled Ameera in the hospital's gender-focused clinic，which sees a wide variety of patients with similar conditions. That helped them navigate the landscape of gender identity，which included providing extensive psychosocial support to the family，and having conversations around hormonal therapy and potential surgeries.

For now，Ameera is a happy，healthy girl，and while she may not choose to identify as a female one day，we'll work to keep up the "healthy" part.

Task 1

Choose the one that best completes the sentence or answers the question according to the text.

1. What was the chief complaint when Ameera saw the family doctor?
   A. Being too anxious.
   B. Stomach pain.
   C. High blood pressure.

2. In children's hospital，Ameera's parents reported the following symptoms except _____ .
   A. feeling nauseous
   B. urinating and feeling thirsty frequently
   C. having high blood pressure

3. High protein levels in her urine test suggested nephrotic syndrome，which explain the following except _____ .
   A. puffy skin around her eyes
   B. high blood pressure

C. the mass near her kidney

4. During the surgery, what shocked the doctors?

    A. Ameera's mass grew out of her left ovary.

    B. Ameera had no right ovary.

    C. Ameera had no uterus.

5. Ameera's missing organs indicated that _____.

    A. she would not be able to bear children

    B. she had Swyer syndrome

    C. she had Denys-Drash syndrome

6. Blood test result showed that _____.

    A. Ameera was chromosomally male

    B. Ameera was chromosomally female

    C. Ameera was neither male nor female

7. What is true about Frasier syndrome?

    A. Patients typically have nephrotic syndrome and gonadoblastoma.

    B. Patients typically have kidney failure.

    C. Patients typically have cancer.

8. So far, the doctors have implemented the following treatment except

    _____.

    A. removing the mass surgically

    B. removing the ovary surgically

    C. blood pressure measurement and water pills

9. Which of the following statement is true?

    A. Ameera's family background required that she must grow up as a female.

    B. Frasier syndrome usually determines one's sexual orientation.

    C. Psychosocial support was provided to Ameera as well as her family.

Task 2

Complete the following case report on Ameera based on the information you obtain from the text.

Age	
Sex	
Growth condition	
Occupation	
Chief complaint	
Other symptoms	
Examinations and laboratory results	
Diagnostic conclusion	
Treatment	
The patient's outcome	
Further proposed treatments	
Patient's present status	

Task 3

Summarize diagnostic and therapeutic procedure of Ameera's disease with the help of the table in task 2.

Reading Aloud

A. 弱化现象（reduction）2

常见功能词的弱化：

1. be 动词——am/əm/或/m/（在元音后），are/ə/或/r/（在元音后），is/s,z/，was /wəz/，were/wə/，been/bɪn/，be/bɪ/

<u>Am</u> I wrong?

Mary<u>'s</u> at home.

2. 助动词——do/də/（在辅音前）或/dʊ/（在元音前），does/dəz，dz/或/s,z/，did /d/，have/həv/、/əv/或/v/（在元音后），has/həz/、/əz/或/s,z/，had/həd/、/əd/或/d/（在元音后）

When <u>do</u> you go to work?

John <u>has</u> found it out.

3. 情态动词——must/məst/，shall/ʃəl/，should/ʃəd/，can/kən/，could/kəd/，will/əl/，would/wəd/、/əd/或/d/

You <u>must</u> leave right now.

He <u>should</u> have arrived.

4. 其他——there be/ðə/，some/səm/，such/sətʃ/，any/əni/，不定式 to/tə/、/ə/（在固定结构中，如 want to/wɑnə/，be going to/gʌnə/，ought to/ɔtə/，have to /hæftə/）

<u>There</u> were some cakes.

We <u>have to</u> leave for the station.

B. Read aloud after the recording.

Perhaps the most important thing people <u>should</u> realize about <u>such</u> epidemics is that the spread of an epidemic in <u>any</u> country endangers the entire human species. In the 1970s，humanity managed to completely eradicate the smallpox virus <u>because</u> all people in <u>all</u> nations were vaccinated against smallpox. If even one country failed to vaccinate its population，it <u>could</u> have endangered the whole of humankind，<u>because</u> as long <u>as</u> the smallpox virus existed <u>and</u> evolved somewhere，it <u>could</u> always spread again everywhere.

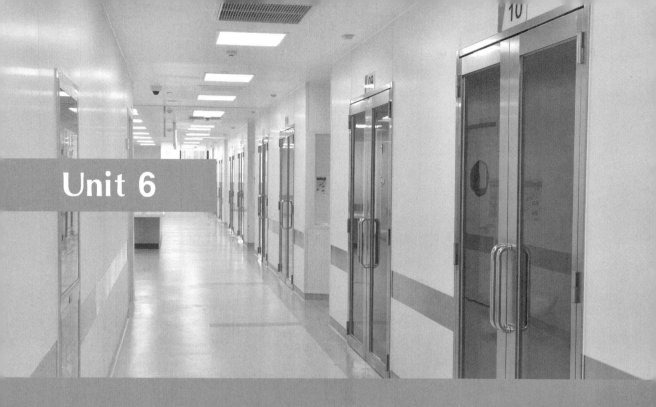

Unit 6

Upon completion of this unit , you will be able to：

- use language of comparison and contrast
- identify key plots by composing interview
- summarize a narration
- learn the pronunciation skill of liaison

✓音视频资源
✓参考答案
✓交流探讨

Text A

chronic [ˈkrɒnɪk] *adj.* 长期的；慢性的

fibromyalgia [faɪbrəʊmaɪˈældʒɪə] *n.* 纤维肌痛；纤维肌痛症

flare-up [ˈfleər ʌp] *n.* 突发；（尤指）复发

pipe up [paɪp ʌp] 开始（大声）讲话

unsolicited [ˌʌnsəˈlɪsɪtɪd] *adj.* 未经要求的；自发的；自我推荐的

Crohn's disease [ˈkrəʊnz dɪˈziːz] 克罗恩病；克罗恩氏病

What I Wish You Knew about My Chronic Illness

By Sophie Kalagas

KERA

Has **Fibromyalgia**

You can't fix it all with yoga and good nutrition! I know there are huge benefits, but the reality for people with fibromyalgia is that there are a lot more challenges than for abled folks. Sometimes going to a yoga class might mean I can't get out of bed for the rest of the week; standing up to cook can cause a **flare-up**. People need to trust us when we communicate our limits, rather than **piping up** with **unsolicited** advice. If a disabled or chronically ill person wants advice, they'll ask for it.

AYAN

Has **Crohn's Disease**

It's frustrating when people say, "I wish I had Crohn's so I could lose weight as fast as you do." When I have a flare-up, I just can't keep anything down. There's a lot of stress about bathrooms and needing to know where the nearest ones are, plus fatigue and exhaustion like no other, and anxiety around food and whether or not it'll make me sick. The unpredictability of it all is really difficult—not knowing whether I'll get sick or end up in hospital sometimes means not being able to plan very far ahead.

BRIDGET

Has **Endometriosis**

Endometriosis is hard on your body, but it's just as **debilitating** for your mental health. I spent six years bouncing between medical professionals before my pain and symptoms were finally taken seriously. With the average diagnosis time between seven and 12 years, it's so easy to feel like nobody cares, and for others to make you feel like it's all in your head. It can also **take quite a toll on** your financial state. Private health insurance, **pelvic** therapy sessions, **acupuncture**, **gynaecologist** and ultrasound appointments, medications ... I don't want to think how much I've spent on endometriosis alone this year!

STEPHANIE

Has **Myalgic Encephalomyelitis**/Chronic Fatigue Syndrome

Being physically unwell and feeling happy aren't mutually exclusive. Being positive and having a good time isn't contradicting my illness. Genuinely smiling through pain has become a skill of mine. It's always nice when people ask how I am before asking about my

endometriosis [ˌɛndoʊˌmɛtrɪˈoʊsɪs] n. 子宫内膜异位
debilitate [dɪˈbɪlɪteɪt] v. (使身心)衰弱,衰竭,虚弱

take a toll on 损害
pelvic [ˈpelvɪk] adj. 靠近骨盆的;骨盆的
acupuncture [ˈækjʊpʌŋktʃə(r)] n. 针刺疗法
gynaecologist [ˌɡaɪnəˈkɒlədʒɪst] n. 妇科医生;妇科学家
myalgic encephalomyelitis [maɪˌældʒɪk enˌsefələʊmaɪəˈlaɪtɪs]肌痛性脑脊髓炎;疲劳症;慢性疲劳综合征

illness. It's usually more fun，too! Having said that，empathy and listening are great，and being understanding is usually more helpful than actually saying，"I understand."

KATHARINE

Has **Multiple Sclerosis** and **Autoimmune Hepatitis**

multiple sclerosis [ˌmʌltɪpl skləˈrəʊsɪs] n. 多发性硬化

autoimmune [ˌɔːtəʊɪˈmjuːn] adj. 自体免疫的

hepatitis [ˌhepəˈtaɪtɪs] n. 肝炎

immune [ɪˈmjuːn] adj. 有免疫力的

Chronic **immune** diseases aren't consistent or predictable. Not only is there a huge variation in how diseases like MS affect different people，the symptoms can also change from week to week and year to year. When I was first diagnosed，I spent a few months only able to walk with a stick—just because I've recovered enough to walk unaided now doesn't mean the disease is "better".

ASHER

Has **Hypermobile Ehlers-Danlos Syndrome** and Related Illnesses

hypermobile Ehlers-Danlos syndrome 超活动性埃勒斯-丹洛斯综合征

rheumatology [ˌruːməˈtɒlədʒɪ] n. 风湿病学

physiotherapy [ˌfɪzɪəʊˈθerəpɪ] n. 理疗；物理治疗

condemn [kənˈdem] v. (通常因道义上的原因而) 谴责，指责

Outpatient waiting lists for specialist services in the public health system are massively long. Public **rheumatology** services at a large hospital in Melbourne have a two-year wait for an initial appointment. **Physiotherapy** is only partially funded on the Medicare Benefits Schedule for five sessions a year，but people with EDS need a session a week on average. We're **condemning** people who live with chronic health conditions to go without diagnosis and adequate management—or go broke paying for management of their condition.

ALANA

Has **Primary Sclerosing Cholangitis** and **Ulcerative Colitis**

I work full-time, I go out with friends, I enjoy a drink from time to time and I try not to focus on my health issues in my day-to-day life (I take my meds, I do my bloods, I get on with it). Because I come across as so healthy to most people, they don't know anything is wrong. This is the case with so many sufferers of chronic illnesses—we all deserve Academy Awards because we're really good at pretending there's nothing wrong. When I do need time off or I'm having a bad health day, people think I'm being dramatic or making things up.

EMILY

Has **Cystic Fibrosis**

What could people do to make my life easier? Stay home if you're unwell and get the flu vaccine! A basic cold may seem like nothing to you, but it can really knock me around and take me months to get rid of. That said, I'm often underestimated, especially by doctors. I recently pushed a 4. 2kg baby out of my **vagina** without any interventions or pain relief, and none of my medical team expected me to be able to because of my limited lung function. I showed them! Everyone with CF is unique, and doctors should

primary sclerosing cholangitis [ˈpraɪmərɪ sklə'rəʊsɪŋ kə'lændʒɪtɪs] 原发性硬化性胆管炎
ulcerative colitis [əl'serətɪv kə'laɪtɪs] 溃疡性结肠炎

cystic fibrosis [ˌsɪstɪk faɪ'brəʊsɪs] n. 囊性纤维变性；囊性纤维化

vagina [və'dʒaɪnə] n. 阴道

understand that most of all.

JASMINE

Has **Polycystic Ovary Syndrome**

Work places need to be more understanding of chronic illnesses relating to women's pain. There seems to be a **rhetoric** that if you're having a painful period，you should just take some pain killers and get on with it，otherwise you're being a bit of a "**hysterical**" woman. But when you can barely walk from the pain and are prescribed strong medicine to help，a little more empathy is really appreciated. Having a flare-up affects my whole body：I have painful periods，my energy levels **fluctuate** with my blood sugar，I get **cystic acne** that affects my confidence，and my mental health suffers.

SANDRA

Has **Rheumatoid Arthritis**

There's not a wide understanding that rheumatoid arthritis is an autoimmune disease，and there are side effects that come with it. People tend to think it's just stiff joints and something only "old" people get. Some of the unexpectedly difficult things I deal with include doing up buttons and opening jar lids. It's the simple things you expect to be able to just do，and when you can't，it can be really frustrating.

polycystic ovary syndrome [ˌpɒliˈsɪstɪkˈəʊvərɪˈsɪndrəum] 多囊卵巢综合征

rhetoric [ˈretərɪk] *n.* 华而不实的言语；花言巧语；修辞技巧；修辞

hysterical [hɪˈsterɪkl] *adj.* 歇斯底里的；情绪狂暴不可抑制的；极其可笑的

fluctuate [ˈflʌktʃueɪt] *v.* 波动

cystic acne [ˈsɪstɪkˈækni] 囊肿性痤疮

rheumatoid arthritis [ˌruːmətɔɪd ɑːˈθraɪtɪs] *n.* 类风湿性关节炎

MICHELLE

Has Endometriosis

Whenever I feel a pain, I don't know if it's my endometriosis or "something to worry about"—a more **sinister** thing. I had an **ovarian cyst** burst once because I ignored it and thought it was endo. That was pretty rubbish. You're never quite sure what's going on with your body, because your baseline isn't zero pain. Sex is always a gamble for me, too. I don't know if it will feel good or hurt. It opens up a lot of communication with my partner, but I really wish it would let me have a good time.

sinister ['sɪnɪstə(r)] *adj.*
邪恶的；险恶的
ovarian cyst [əʊ'veərɪən sɪst]卵巢囊肿

Task 1

Come up with 10 questions about the text. The questions can be about the main idea or important details of the story. They can also be inference drawn from the text or lessons learned.

Model question:

1. What kind of advice would Kera not want to hear from others? Why?

2. _____

3. _____

4. _____

5. _____

6. _____

7. _____

8. _____

9. _____

10. _____

Task 2

Answer the questions in Task 1.

Model question & answer：

1. What kind of advice would Kera not want to hear from others? Why?

Answer：Advice like "You should practice yoga and get good nutrition. They are helpful for your health.", because having yoga class might hurt and standing up to cook can cause a flare-up.

2. _____

_____

_____

_____

3. _____

_____

_____

_____

4. _____

_____

_____

_____

5. _____

_____

6. _____

7. _____

8. _____

9. _____

10. _____

_____

_____

_____

Task 3

Fill in the following table with chief information you learn about the chronic disease patients.

Names	Diseases	Main challenges	Others can help by ...
Kera	fibromyalgia	People do not show empathy and give undesirable advice.	Trying to understand the patients.
Ayan			
Bridget		1. It takes quite a few years of struggle just to diagnose this disease. 2. 3.	
Stephanie			
Katharine			
Asher			
Alana			
Emily			
Jasmine			
Sandra			
Michelle			

Text B

What Can We Learn From Amish People?

By Jeffrey Kluger

These **devout** communities, **predominantly** located in Pennsylvania, Ohio and Indiana, go without cars, TVS, computers, phones or even the electricity needed to run so much of 21st century **gadgetry**. But what researchers who have studied them have found is what the Amish have a **surplus** of: good health in late life. The average American **life expectancy** is currently just under 79 years. Back in 1900, it was only 47, but for early-20th century Amish it was already greater than 70. Over the decades, most Americans have caught up in overall life expectancy, but the Amish still have a significant **edge** in late-life health, with lower rates of cancer, cardiovascular disease, diabetes and more. So how do they do it?

Start with lifestyle. Amish communities are **agrarian**, with no modern farm equipment, meaning all the work has to be done by hand. In 2004, the American College of Sports Medicine fitted Amish volunteers with **pedometers** to determine how much physical activity they performed. The results were dramatic. Amish men took 18,425 steps a day and

devout [dɪˈvaʊt] *adj.* 笃信宗教的;虔诚的
predominantly [prɪˈdɒmɪnəntlɪ] *adv.* 主要地;多数情况下
gadgetry [ˈgædʒɪtrɪ] *n.* (统称)小器具,小装置
surplus [ˈsɜːpləs] *n.* 剩余;盈余
life expectancy 预期寿命

edge [edʒ] *n.* 优势

agrarian [əˈgreərɪən] *adj.* 农业的;土地的

pedometer [pɪˈdɒmɪtə(r)] *n.* 计步器

women 14,196 steps, compared with non-Amish people who are encouraged by doctors to shoot for at least 10,000 steps—and typically fail. Including other forms of manual labor—lifting, chopping, sowing, planting—the Amish are six times as active as a random sample of people from 12 countries.

One result of this is that only about 4% of Amish people are obese, compared with 36.5% of the overall US population. Amish children are about one-third as likely as non-Amish to be obese, according to a 2012 study in PLoS One. This means 50% lower rates of Type 2 diabetes.

The near absence of tobacco in the Amish community—some men do smoke cigars—results in a 63% lower rate of tobacco-related cancers, according to a 2004 study of Ohio's Amish population. The Amish also had rates of all cancers that were 40% lower than the rest of the Ohio population.

attributable [ə'trɪbjətəbl] *adj*. 可归因于；可能由于

gravy ['greɪvɪ] *n*. （调味）肉汁

carb [kɑːb] *n*. 淀粉质食物；高碳水化合物食物

Cardiovascular disease is one area in which the Amish don't have an edge, with blood-pressure and heart-disease rates slightly higher than those of other populations. Some of this might be **attributable** to the Amish diet, which is heavy on pancakes, eggs and sausage for breakfast; and meat, potatoes, **gravy** and bread for dinner. Working the farm can burn off those calories, but all the fat and salt and **carbs** still take a toll.

The most powerful weapon in the Amish long-life

arsenal, however, may be genes. The Amish population in the US is about 318,000, **descended from** just 200 families that immigrated in the 1700s. They mostly marry within their own communities, which means the genes that existed when their ancestors got to America have remained. That can be a dangerous thing if bad genes are hidden in the mix but a good thing if the genes are sound. While no community is without genetic problems, the Amish seem to have gotten a **lucky draw**.

In a study released last November, researchers at Northwestern University announced the discovery of a gene in an Amish community that seemed to be associated with an average life span 10% longer than that of people without the gene. The long-lived **subjects** also had 10% longer **telomeres**—the caps at the end of chromosomes that shorten over time and drive the aging process. The gene, known as PAI-1, is linked not only to slower aging but also to better **insulin** levels and better blood pressure and **arterial** flexibility.

Not all Amish have the PAI-1 mutation; it has been found so far in just one community in Indiana. But those who do carry it have an additional edge over and above the one they have simply from being born Amish.

While much of the Amish advantage is unique to the Amish themselves, there is one long-life lesson they can teach everyone else. Almost all elderly people

arsenal [ˈɑːsənl] *n.* 武器;兵工厂;宝库

be descended from 是某人的后裔

lucky draw 幸运抽奖

subject [ˈsʌbdʒɪkt] *n.* 研究对象;实验对象

telomere [ˈtɛləmɪr] 端粒;染色体端粒;染色体末端

insulin [ˈɪnsjəlɪn] *n.* 胰岛素

arterial [ɑːˈtɪərɪəl] *adj.* 动脉的

dividend ［'dɪvɪdend］ *n.*
红利

trump ［trʌmp］ *v.* 赢；胜
过；打败

in the Amish community are cared for at home，by relatives. This isn't always realistic or possible in the non-Amish world，but when it is，it pays huge health **dividends**. The PLoS One study estimated that aging in place has the same longevity benefits as quitting smoking. In all communities，it seems，the power of family may **trump** the power of medicine.

Task 1

The author of this article makes comparison and contrast between Amish people and others. For example：

Amish men took 18,425 steps a day and women 14,196 steps，compared with non-Amish people who are encouraged by doctors to shoot for at least 10,000 steps—and typically fail.

The following words and expressions are often used to signal comparison and contrast：

Comparison	Contrast
similarly	on the other hand
likewise	by contrast
both	however
same	while
resemble	although
nor	different from
comparable	unlike
similar to	rather than
in the same way	instead (of)

The following sentences are taken from the text. All the signpost language indicating comparison and contrast has been removed. Complete the sentences and then compare your answers with the original sentences.

1. The average American life expectancy is currently just under 79 years. Back in 1900, it was only 47, _____ for early-20th century Amish it was already greater than 70.

2. Including other forms of manual labor—lifting, chopping, sowing, planting—the Amish are six _____ as active as a random sample of people from 12 countries.

3. One result of this is that only about 4% of Amish people are obese, _____ 36.5% of the overall US population.

4. Amish children are about one-third as likely as non-Amish to be obese, according to a 2012 study in PLoS One. This means 50% _____ rates of Type 2 diabetes.

5. The Amish also had rates of all cancers that were 40% _____ the rest of the Ohio population.

6. Cardiovascular disease is one area in which the Amish don't have an edge, with blood-pressure and heart-disease rates slightly _____ than those of other populations.

7. That can be a dangerous thing if bad genes are hidden in the mix _____ a good thing if the genes are sound.

8. _____ no community is without genetic problems, the Amish seem to have gotten a lucky draw.

Task 2

The English Broadcasting Radio in your school is going to hold an interview program about healthy life style. An expert of Amish people research, Professor Lee, is invited to the program. What questions would you ask if you were the interviewer? How would you answer them if you were the interviewee?

Q: _____

A: _____

_____

Q:＿＿＿＿＿＿＿＿＿＿＿＿＿＿＿＿＿＿＿＿＿＿＿＿＿

A:＿＿＿＿＿＿＿＿＿＿＿＿＿＿＿＿＿＿＿＿＿＿＿＿＿

＿＿＿＿＿＿＿＿＿＿＿＿＿＿＿＿＿＿＿＿＿＿＿＿＿＿＿

Q:＿＿＿＿＿＿＿＿＿＿＿＿＿＿＿＿＿＿＿＿＿＿＿＿＿

A:＿＿＿＿＿＿＿＿＿＿＿＿＿＿＿＿＿＿＿＿＿＿＿＿＿

＿＿＿＿＿＿＿＿＿＿＿＿＿＿＿＿＿＿＿＿＿＿＿＿＿＿＿

Q:＿＿＿＿＿＿＿＿＿＿＿＿＿＿＿＿＿＿＿＿＿＿＿＿＿

A:＿＿＿＿＿＿＿＿＿＿＿＿＿＿＿＿＿＿＿＿＿＿＿＿＿

＿＿＿＿＿＿＿＿＿＿＿＿＿＿＿＿＿＿＿＿＿＿＿＿＿＿＿

Q:＿＿＿＿＿＿＿＿＿＿＿＿＿＿＿＿＿＿＿＿＿＿＿＿＿

A:＿＿＿＿＿＿＿＿＿＿＿＿＿＿＿＿＿＿＿＿＿＿＿＿＿

＿＿＿＿＿＿＿＿＿＿＿＿＿＿＿＿＿＿＿＿＿＿＿＿＿＿＿

Q:＿＿＿＿＿＿＿＿＿＿＿＿＿＿＿＿＿＿＿＿＿＿＿＿＿

A:＿＿＿＿＿＿＿＿＿＿＿＿＿＿＿＿＿＿＿＿＿＿＿＿＿

＿＿＿＿＿＿＿＿＿＿＿＿＿＿＿＿＿＿＿＿＿＿＿＿＿＿＿

Q:＿＿＿＿＿＿＿＿＿＿＿＿＿＿＿＿＿＿＿＿＿＿＿＿＿

A:＿＿＿＿＿＿＿＿＿＿＿＿＿＿＿＿＿＿＿＿＿＿＿＿＿

＿＿＿＿＿＿＿＿＿＿＿＿＿＿＿＿＿＿＿＿＿＿＿＿＿＿＿

Task 3

Think of your lifestyle. What do you learn from Amish people to improve your way of life?

Reading Aloud

A. 连读(liaison)1——辅元连读

辅元连读(C+V)是指同一语句中以辅音结尾和以元音或半元音开头的两个单词，滑读时听起来好像在结尾的辅音和开头的元音之间自然连接上了。辅元连读可以分为以下两种情况：

1. 辅元连读(C+V)：语句中以辅音结尾和以元音开头的两个单词在滑读中听起来好像自然连接上了。

Look～up   think～about   believe～in   some～apples
one～of～us   dead～or alive   where is～it

2. 辅半连读(C+/j/)：语句中以辅音结尾和以半元音/j/开头的两个单词在滑读中听起来好像自然连接上了。其中/s/+/j/听起来很像/ʃ/，/z/+/j/听起来很像/ʒ/，/t/+/j/听起来很像/tʃ/，/d/和/j/听起来很像/dʒ/。

miss～you   bless～you   lose～you   as～usual
meet～you   last～year   did～you   called～you

B. Read aloud after the recording.

1. Cardiovascular disease is one～area in which the Amish don't have～an～edge.

2. People with EDS need～a session～a week～on～average.

3. Everyone with CF～is unique，and doctors should～understand that most～of～all.

4. While much～of the Amish～advantage～is unique to the Amish themselves，there～is one long-life lesson they can teach～everyone～else.

5. When～I do need time～off or I'm having～a bad health day，people think I'm being dramatic～or making things～up.

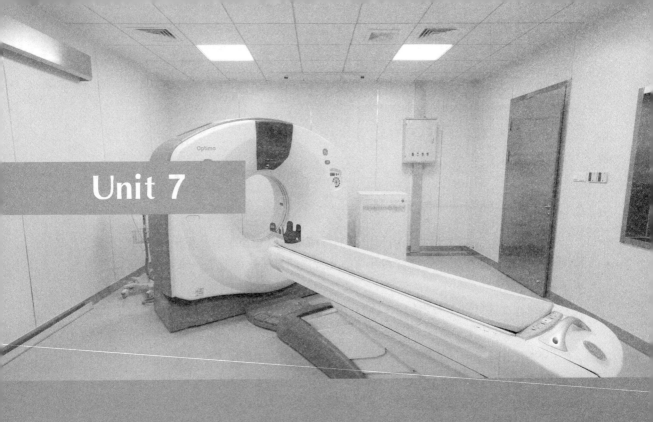

Unit 7

Upon completion of this unit，you will be able to：

- sort out main ideas of an expository writing
- illustrate steps of a procedure
- identify key plots by composing interview
- organize language with cause-effect relationship
- draw a mind map to clarify expository writing
- learn the pronunciation skill of liaison

✓音视频资源
✓参考答案
✓交流探讨

Text A

Find Peace Anytime，Anyplace

[Meditation is simpler than it sounds. Follow these directions from a skeptic who tried and liked it.]

By Dan Harris and Jeffrey Warren with Carlye Adler

If you had told me as recently as a few years ago that I would someday become a traveling **evangelist** for meditation，I would have coughed my beer up through my nose.

In 2004，I had a panic attack at work. Unfortunately for me，that meant in front of millions of people，as I was delivering the news，live，on ABC's Good Morning America. In the wake of my nationally televised **freak-out**，I learned that I had undiagnosed depression. For months，I'd been having trouble getting out of bed in the morning and felt as if I had a permanent low-grade fever.

The panic attack ultimately led me to embrace a practice I had always dismissed as ridiculous. For most of my life，to the extent that I'd ever even considered meditation，I ranked it right alongside **aura** readings and Enya. Further，I figured my racing type A mind was way too busy to ever be able to **commune with** the

meditation [ˌmedɪˈteɪʃn] *n*. 冥想；沉思

evangelist [ɪˈvændʒəlɪst] *n*. (基督教)布道者

freak-out [friːk aʊt]发狂

aura [ˈɔːrə] *n*. 气氛；氛围；气质

commune with [ˈkɒmjuːn wɪð]交流；谈心；与……谈心

cosmos ['kɒzmɒs] n. 宇宙

hormone cortisol
['hɔːmoʊn 'kɔrtɪˌsɔl] 皮质醇；激素皮质醇
atrophy ['ætrəfɪ] n. 萎缩
mitigate ['mɪtɪgeɪt] v. 减轻；缓和

neuroscience
['njʊərəʊsaɪəns] n. 神经科学

resilience [rɪ'zɪlɪəns] n. 快速恢复的能力；适应力；还原能力；弹力

pretzel ['pretsl] n. 椒盐卷饼

cosmos. And anyway, if I got too happy, it would probably render me completely ineffective at my hyper-competitive job.

Two things changed my mind. The first was the science. In recent years, there has been an explosion of research into meditation, which has been shown to reduce blood pressure, boost recovery after your body releases the stress **hormone cortisol**, strengthen the immune system, slow age-related **atrophy** of the brain, and **mitigate** the symptoms of depression and anxiety. Studies also show meditation can reduce violence in prisons, increase productivity in the workplace, and improve both the behavior and the grades of schoolchildren.

Things really get interesting when you look at the **neuroscience**. In recent years, researchers have been peering into the heads of mediators, and they've found that the practice can rewire key parts of the brain involved with self-awareness, compassion, and **resilience**. One study from the Harvard Gazette found that just eight weeks of meditation resulted in measurable decreases in gray matter density in the area of the brain associated with stress.

The second thing that changed my mind about meditation is that it does not necessarily entail a lot of the "weird" stuff I feared it might. Contrary to popular belief, meditation does not have to involve folding yourself into a **pretzel**, joining a group, or wearing special outfits. The word meditation is a little bit like the word sports; there are hundreds of varieties. The type of meditation discussed here is called mindfulness meditation，which is derived from **Buddhism** but does not require adopting a belief system or declaring oneself to be a Buddhist.

> Buddhism ['bʊdɪzəm] *n.* 佛教

I began my practice slowly，with just five to ten minutes a day，which is what I recommend everyone aim for at the start（Frankly, if you find time for even one minute a day，you can count that as a win）.

The practice does get easier the longer you keep at it，but even after doing it for years，I get lost all the time. Here's a random sample of my mental chatter during a typical session：

In.

Out.

Man，I am feeling **antsy**. What's the **Yiddish** term my grandmother used to use for that? Shpilkes. Right.

> antsy ['æntsɪ] *adj.* 烦躁的；坐立不安的
> Yiddish ['jɪdɪʃ] *n.* 意第绪语，依地语
> ointment ['ɔɪntmənt] *n.* 药膏；软膏；油膏

Words that always make me giggle：**ointment**, pianist.

Wait，what? Come on，man. Back to the breath.

In.

Out.

Likes：baked goods.

> fedora [fɪ'dɔːrə] *n.* 浅顶卷檐软呢帽
> accordion [ə'kɔːdɪən] *n.* 手风琴

Dislikes：**fedoras**，dream sequences, that part in techno songs where the French **accordion** kicks in.

Dude. Come. On.

In.

Out.

In.

papal nuncio ['peɪpl 'nʌnsɪəʊ] 教廷大使

Alternative jobs: **papal nuncio**, interpretive dancer, working double time on the seduction line ...

You get the idea.

To give you a sense of exactly how simple it is, here are the three-step instructions for beginning meditation.

Sit comfortably. It's best to have your spine reasonably straight, which may help prevent an involuntary nap. If you want to sit cross-legged on the floor, go for it. If not, just sit in a chair, as I do. You can close your eyes or, if you prefer, leave them open and adjust your gaze to a neutral point on the ground.

prominent ['prɒmɪnənt] adj. 显眼的；显著的；突出的
nostril ['nɒstrəl] n. 鼻孔

Bring your full attention to the feeling of your breath coming in and out. Pick a spot where it's most **prominent**: your chest, your belly, or your **nostrils**. You're not thinking about your breath; you're just feeling the physical sensations. To help maintain focus, make a quiet mental note on each in breath and out breath, like "in" and "out."

escort ['eskɔːt] v. 护卫；护送

Every time you catch yourself wandering, **escort** your attention back to the breath. This third step is the key. As soon as you try to focus on your breath, you'll start having all sorts of random thoughts，such as：What's for lunch? Do I need a haircut? What was Casper the Friendly Ghost before he died? Who was the Susan after whom they named the lazy Susan，and how did she feel about it? This is totally normal. The whole game is to notice when you're distracted and begin again. And again. And again. It is like a **biceps** curl for the brain. It is also a **radical** act：You're breaking a lifetime's habit of walking around in a fog of **rumination** and projection，and focusing on what's happening right now.

People assume they can never meditate because they can't stop thinking. I cannot say this enough：The goal is not to clear your mind but to focus your mind—for a few **nanoseconds** at a time—and whenever you become distracted，just start again. Getting lost and starting over is not failing at meditation. It is succeeding.

I have been meditating for eight years，and I am still plenty ambitious. However，these days I'm not as sweaty，agitated，and unpleasant about it as I used to be. Meditation has helped me sort out my useless **rumination** from what I call **constructive anguish**.

I have learned that the less **enchanted** you are by the voice in your head，the more you can make room for entirely new thoughts and feelings to emerge. It has enabled me to take even more delight in my work，my wife，and our son，Alexander，who **suffuses** me

biceps [ˈbaɪseps] *n.* 二头肌

radical [ˈrædɪkl] *adj.* 根本的；彻底的；完全的

rumination [ˌruːmɪˈneɪʃn] *n.* 沉思；认真考虑

nanosecond [ˈnænəʊsekənd] *n.* 毫微秒；十亿分之一秒

constructive [kənˈstrʌktɪv] *adj.* 建设性的；有助益的；积极的

anguish [ˈæŋgwɪʃ] *n.* 剧痛；极度痛苦；苦恼

enchanted [ɪnˈtʃɑːntɪd] *adj.* 中魔法的；着了魔的；狂喜的

suffuse [səˈfjuːz] *v.* 布满；弥漫于；充满

nugget ['nʌgɪt] n. 小圆块

macerate ['mæsəreɪt] v. 把(食物等)浸软

in thrall [ɪn θrɔːl] 受奴役

aversion [ə'vɜːʃn] n. 厌恶；憎恶

ineffable [ɪn'efəbl] adj. (美好得)难以形容的，不可言喻的

unclench [ʌn'klentʃ] v. (使)松开；松开

ego ['iːgəʊ] n. 自我价值感；自我

with warmth whether he's offering me a chicken **nugget** or wiping **macerated** muffin on my sleeve. I am less **in thrall** to my desires and **aversions**, which has given me a wider perspective and, at times, a taste of a deep, **ineffable unclenching**. In sum, meditation empowers you to tap into what lies beneath or beyond the **ego**. Call it creativity. Call it your innate wisdom. Some people call it your heart.

Task 1

Complete the chart about the positive effects of meditation upon physical and mental health.

To benefit physical health, meditation can ...	To benefit mental health, meditation can ...
reduce _____ .	mitigate the symptoms of _____ and _____ .
boost _____ after the body releases the _____ .	reduce _____ in prisons; increase ____ _____ in the workplace.
strengthen the _____ .	improve both the _____ and the _____ of schoolchildren.
slow _____ of the brain.	rewire key parts of the brain involved with _____ , _____ , and _____ .
	result in decreases in _____ in the area of the brain associated with stress.

Task 2

Try to teach your friends about the three steps of meditation while showing the practice yourself. How do you instruct the others? Complete the following script of what you say.

Well guys, meditation is pretty simple. Here is how you do it. To begin with,

_____

_____

_____

Next, _____

_____

_____

_____

Every time you catch yourself wandering, _____

_____

_____

Maybe you think you can't stop wandering, _____

_____

_____

_____

Task 3

Suppose there is a TV interview with the narrator in this article about meditation. What questions would you ask if you were the interviewer? How would you answer them if you were the interviewee?

Question: Hello, Mr. Adler. How long have you been practicing meditation?

Answer: I have been mediating for eight years. _____

Q: _____

A: _____

Q: _____

A: _____

Q: _____

A: _____

Q: _____

A: _____

Q: _____

A: _____

Text B

A Day in the Life of Your Skin

By Teresa Dumain

Three alarm snoozes, a leg **scratch**, and 14 eye rubs later, you roll out of bed and **plod** into the kitchen to make coffee. You're totally entitled to take it slow after a tough week, but I wish you'd rub me less. I'm thinnest around your eyes. At only about 0. 05 mm thick—half the thickness of computer paper—I get tiny tears in **capillaries** from all that **manhandling**, making me look discolored and older. Oy, make that 15 eye rubs.

My Favorite Shower Routine

Adequately caffeinated, you head to the bathroom to shower. As you wait for the water to warm, you give me a good scratch and then another. It always happens more this time of year. The dry air sucks moisture out through my top layer, which makes me irritated. Literally.

Dryness triggers an inflammatory response: Immune cells as well as **pro-inflammatory** proteins and other **enzymes** go wild, activating itch **receptors** that send signals to your brain. The result: your fingernails

---

scratch [skrætʃ] n. 搔痒
plod [plɒd] v. 艰难地行走;吃力地行进

capillary [kə'pɪlərɪ] n. 毛细血管
manhandle ['mænhændl] v. (粗暴地)推搡,拉扯,对待

pro-inflammatory [prəʊ ɪn'flæmətrɪ] adj. 促炎性的;致发炎的;促发炎的
enzyme ['enzaɪm] n. 酶
receptor [rɪ'septə(r)] n. 感受器;受体

refire [rɪˈfaɪə(r)] v. 再点燃

vicious circle [ˌvɪʃəs ˈsɜːkl] 恶性循环

soothe [suːð] v. 安慰；抚慰

lubricate [ˈluːbrɪkeɪt] v. 给……上润滑油；上油于

debris [ˈdebriː] n. 残骸；碎片

clog [klɒg] v. (使)阻塞，堵塞

pore [pɔː(r)] n. (皮肤上的)毛孔

scrub [skrʌb] v. 擦洗；刷洗

moisturize [ˈmɔɪstʃəraɪz] v. 使皮肤湿润

slop [slɒp] v. 倒出

petroleum [pəˈtrəʊliəm] n. 石油；原油

ceramide [səˈræmaɪd] n. 天然保湿因子

molecule [ˈmɒlɪkjuːl] n. 分子

dewy [ˈdjuːɪ] adj. 露水打湿的；带露水的

raking across me (not so gently, I might add). I know it feels good for a second—scratching may engage pleasure and reward centers in the brain. But if you keep at it, I'll get even more inflamed, which will cause those itch receptors to **refire**. And a **vicious circle** continues. All. Winter. Long.

As much as you want to linger under the **soothing** stream of water, I beg you to stop after ten minutes. Long, hot showers strip away my natural oils, as do soapy cleansers. The fact that you switched to a gentle, soap-free body wash for this time of year is perfect—it'll get rid of dirt but leave some oils to help me stay **lubricated**. I'm also grateful that you skipped washing your face this morning. If I could make a PSA for this, I would: Ladies, you don't need to wash your face twice a day(especially if you have dry skin). One cleansing at night gets rid of the **debris** that can **clog** my **pores**. **Scrubbing** again in the morning may remove too much oil.

After a quick pat-down, you dip into that new jar of **moisturizing** ointment and start **slopping** it on while I'm still damp. Ahhhh. Hello, happy place. This is exactly what I need—it's thick and **petroleum**-based and contains **ceramides**. These lipids occur naturally in my top layer, but this time of year, I welcome an extra dose. They trap water **molecules** to help me stay smooth and **dewy**.

I'm Tougher than I Look

You're always doing things to "boost your **immunity**." If only you knew that I'm your first line of defense against **germs**! All three of my layers—my outer **epidermis**, thickest middle **dermis**, and bottom fatty layer—protect against invading **bacteria**, **fungi**, and other undesirables. That's also why I'm lucky you're so **diligent** about moisturizing. If my outer layer gets too dry, tiny cracks can develop, which leaves me looking scaly—and you more **prone to** skin infections and inflammation.

But if I'm **intact**, I must say, I do my job well. Like right now. You decide to take your kids to story time at the bookstore—talk about a germ zone. But I handily **thwart** the bugs you encounter: **lurking** along the escalator and spread all over the toys and board books in the kiddie section. I may feel soft, but don't be fooled. I'm as tough as nails. My epidermal cells create a dry, acidic environment that's hostile to bacteria. These cells also have a secret weapon: **tentacle**-like **appendages** that seek and destroy germs. And they secrete enzymes that help **foil** unwanted visitors.

When you bump into a table display, it's my innermost layer of fat and **collagen** cells that absorbs the shock and protects your inner organs, and it's my blood vessels that bear the brunt of the jolt. Hip-check the table hard enough, and it'll break the capillaries

immunity [ɪˈmjuːnətɪ] *n.* 免疫力

germ [dʒɜːm] *n.* 微生物；细菌；病菌

epidermis [ˌepɪˈdɜːmɪs] *n.* 表皮

dermis [ˈdɜːmɪs] *n.* 真皮

bacteria [bækˈtɪərɪə] *n.* 细菌

fungi [ˈfʌŋɡaɪ] *v.* (fungus 的复数)真菌；霉菌

diligent [ˈdɪlɪdʒənt] *adj.* 孜孜不倦的；勤勉的

be prone to 易于……的

intact [ɪnˈtækt] *adj.* 完好无损；完整

thwart [θwɔːt] *v.* 阻止；阻挠

lurk [lɜːk] *v.* 埋伏，潜伏

tentacle [ˈtentəkl] *n.* 触角；触手

appendage [əˈpendɪdʒ] *n.* 附加物；附属物

foil [fɔɪl] *v.* 挫败，阻止

collagen [ˈkɒlədʒən] *n.* 胶原蛋白

unsightly [ʌn'saɪtlɪ] *adj.* 难看的；不雅观的

hemoglobin [ˌhiːməʊ'gləʊbɪn] *n.* 血红蛋白

bruise [bruːz] *n.* 青肿；瘀伤

near my top layer, causing blood to leak into the surrounding tissue and form that **unsightly** mark. As the **hemoglobin** in the blood—which gives the **bruise** its purplish color—breaks down over time, the bruise turns Technicolor, fading to greenish yellow and then golden brown. Soon enough, I'll be back to normal as white blood cells finish repairing the damage.

My Big Winter Worry

abrasive [ə'breɪsɪv] *adj.* 研磨的；生硬粗暴的

sanitize ['sænɪtaɪz] *v.* 净化

squirt [skwɜːt] *v.* 喷

I'm glad you layered a cotton T-shirt under your sweater, the wool is a little **abrasive**. (It can even trigger a rash if I'm feeling particularly sensitive.) And thank goodness for your gloves. That **sanitizing** gel you **squirted** on after leaving the bookstore strips my natural oils. The gloves block the harsh outdoor air and help trap whatever moisture I have left.

ultraviolet rays [ˌʌltrə'vaɪələt 'reɪz] 紫外线

cringe [krɪndʒ] *v.* 感到尴尬不安；觉得难为情

saggy ['sægi] *adj.* 松垂的；松弛耷拉的

But if I can complain for a sec, I don't get why you skipped the face lotion with SPF 30 this morning. You moisturize anyway; it can't get any easier. Even applying a face powder with SPF would be better than nothing. Maybe you don't realize that as long as it's daylight, those **ultraviolet rays** are around, regardless of the weather. In winter, there can be up to twice as many UVA rays as UVB—these penetrate deep into me and contribute to cancer and most of the problems you see in your skin: the wrinkles that make you **cringe**, the dark spots on your hands, and the **saggy** neck you hate in photos. It makes me, well, crawl when you don't use sunscreen religiously.

Feed Me Well

As you pass your favorite restaurant on your way home, you decide to treat the kids to an early dinner. Burger and fries for them; **salmon** and broccoli for you. You know this choice is smart for your waistline, but it does me good as well. The fish is packed with omega-3s, which can help **replenish** my natural oils as well as fight inflammation; the broccoli has loads of vitamin C, which my cells require to make collagen, a protein that makes me firm and supple. And thanks for skipping dessert! Sugar molecules bind to my proteins, which compromises the fibers that keep me **taut**. (Translation: wrinkles.)

Trust Me, Beauty Sleep Is Real

You're turning in early tonight, which is exactly what I need to do my repair work. All day long, I've been making fresh new cells and pushing up dead ones to the top to be **sloughed** off. This renewal process speeds up during deep sleep. In roughly a month, my top layer will be fully **regenerated. Humidifier** on? Check Face washed? Yup. Another **rubdown** with ointment? Love you. Now I just hope the kids let you sleep through the night. People who get uninterrupted, high-quality sleep show half as many signs of aging as poor sleepers. Good sleepers have fewer fine lines, better **elasticity**, and more even tone. I'll also recover more efficiently from stressors, and let's face it: I'll look more attractive. I'm the first one

salmon ['sæmən] *n.* 鲑鱼

replenish [rɪ'plenɪʃ] *v.* 补充

taut [tɔːt] *adj.* 拉紧的；绷紧的

slough [slaʊ] *v.* 蜕（皮）；使脱落
regenerate [rɪ'dʒenəreɪt] *v.* 再生；使再生
humidifier [hjuː'mɪdɪfaɪə(r)] *n.* 加湿器；增湿器
rubdown ['rʌbˌdaʊn] *n.* 磨平

elasticity [ˌiːlæ'stɪsətɪ] *n.* 弹性；弹力

to say that beauty is supposed to be more than skin-deep. But I also know that when I'm healthy, you feel beautiful—and that's worth all my efforts.

Task 1

Fill in the following table with 10 pairs of cause-effect relationship. Then make sentences with cause-effect signal words, such as:

because   since   due to   caused by   result from/in   lead to   therefore consequently   thus   as a result   the outcome   on that account

Cause	Effect
Skin around the eyes gets tiny tears in capillaries from rub.	The skin looks discolored and older.

Task 2

Base on the text, draw a mind map.

Task 3

Introduce skin care to others with the help of the mind map you have drawn.

Reading Aloud

A. 连读(liaison)2——元元连读

元元连读(V+V)是指同一语句中的以元音结尾和以元音开头的两个单词在滑读中听起来好像在结尾的元音和开头的元音之间多了一个语音音素。元元连读有以下情形：

1. Linking/j/：语句中以/ɪ/、/iː/、/e/、/eɪ/、/aɪ/、/ɔɪ/结尾和以元音开头的两个单词在滑读中听起来好像在这两个元音之间多了一个半元音/j/。

we～agree	my～uncle	hurry～up	see～us
the toy～is	they～already	try～it	give me～a call

2. Linking/w/：语句中以/u/、/uː/、/əʊ/、/aʊ/结尾和以元音开头的两个单词在滑读中听起来好像在这两个元音之间多了一个半元音/w/。

you～ask	go～over	too～upset	do～I
go～out	now～and then	how～often	How～are you?

B. Read aloud after the recording.

1. Three～alarm snoozes, a leg scratch, and 14 eye rubs later, you roll out of bed and plod into the kitchen to make coffee.

2. At only～about 0.05 mm thick—half the thickness of computer paper—I get tiny tears in capillaries from all that manhandling.

3. The dry～air sucks moisture out through my top layer, which makes me～irritated.

4. You don't need to wash your face twice a day (especially～if you have dry skin).

5. It's my～innermost layer of fat and collagen cells that absorbs the shock and protects your inner organs.

6. It can't get any～easier.

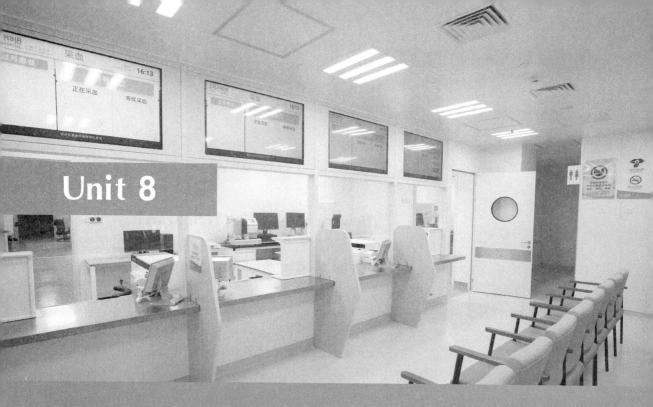

Unit 8

Upon completion of this unit，you will be able to：

- sort out sequence of a narration
- retell the story with the help of connectives given
- draw a mind map to clarify text's main ideas
- deliver a presentation about the text
- learn the pronunciation skill of liaison

✓音视频资源
✓参考答案
✓交流探讨

Text A

Beware of Medical Web Searches

〔You can find good information，but there's a lot more bad.〕

By Zeynep Tufekci

When a sharp chest pain woke me up around 3 a.m.，I had the obvious question：Was this truly panic-worthy？ This had never happened to me before，and I'm in fairly good health—but I had lost one parent to a sudden，early death that may have been a **cardiac** event（we never learned for sure）.

I may have the word "doctor" in my title，but I'm not that kind of doctor. I thought about dialing 911，but then I noticed that … well，the pain was on the right side of my chest rather than the left. My breathing wasn't labored. My heart wasn't pounding. So like millions before me，I Googled my symptoms. On top of the screen was an article entitled "16 Causes of Right Side Chest Pain." Bingo，I thought—except it was an ad. I moved on to the actual search results，which were headlined "17 Causes of Pain in the Right Side of the Chest" and "26 Causes of Chest Pain & Tightness." When I got to "3 Types of Chest Pain That Won't Kill You，" I started wondering：What were all

cardiac〔'kɑːdɪæk〕*adj*. 心脏的；心脏病的

these **bizarre** articles?

Suddenly, my medically useless **doctorate** seemed to be more and more relevant. The titles were about gaming Google's search **algorithm** to grab people's attention at their vulnerable moments. This is called search-engine **optimization**, or SEO: the art and science of engineering for higher **placement** in Google search results and getting people to click on the links.

Unlike a lot of "medical information" online, SEO itself is **steep** in the scientific method, which shows that this number-heavy format plays to a human **cognitive** bias called stand-out. We notice things that stand out—like oddly precise numbers. When I was a child in Turkey, my grandmother loved various over-the-counter remedies for maladies from the most minor to the serious, and many of them contained **menthol**. Menthol may not always have been the active ingredient, but it gave a soothing, medicinal aura to the lotions and rubs that filled her cupboard. Similarly, these odd, specific numbers add a scientific aura to the headlines.

I still needed information, though, so I clicked on a result from WebMD. I had seen that site before, and it didn't seem like it was **quackery**. I was barely a paragraph or two in when I noticed links about lung cancer symptoms. Huh? Lung cancer often causes no pain until its later stages. Then I realized that the information about lung cancer was an ad, but the "ad"

bizarre [bɪˈzɑː(r)] adj. 极其怪诞的;异乎寻常的

doctorate [ˈdɒktərət] n. 博士学位

algorithm [ˈælɡərɪðəm] n. 算法;计算程序

optimization [ˌɒptɪmaɪˈzeɪʃn] n. 最佳(优)化;优选法

placement [ˈpleɪsmənt] n. 安置,放置

steep [stiːp] v. 泡;浸;使……充满

cognitive [ˈkɒɡnətɪv] adj. 认知的;感知的;认识的

menthol [ˈmenθɒl] n. 薄荷醇

quackery [ˈkwækəri] n. 江湖医术;庸医行径

notation was barely noticeable. During an emergency is obviously not the best time to scare people into clicking links for unlikely diseases. Indeed，if you clicked on these "lung cancer symptoms," the browser took you eventually to a site advertising a lung cancer medication from Merck. Ugh.

Using inappropriate screenings and symptoms to advertise for drugs is not new at all. As early as 2010，WebMD had gotten in hot water for a depression screener consisting of 10 questions that，no matter how you answered，spat out the same answer："You may be at risk for major depression." You can almost smell the **legalese**：we all may be at risk for major depression anyway. No need for a quiz sponsored by Eli Lilly，a company that just happens to manufacture the **antidepressant Cymbalta**.

Having medical information online be financed by advertisers or **pharmaceutical** companies—or supplement manufacturers—is certainly not healthy. They often have an **incentive** to scare us. It's a lose-lose situation. Sometimes we do need to be worried and seek medical care. Other times its just **fearmongering** for clicks. But who can tell when one is in crisis?

Finally，I looked up whether my own university had a health information site. Sure enough，there was a site with precise answers for exactly my question，the first statement being that "**pinpoint** chest pain" like

legalese［ˌliːɡəˈliːz］n. （深奥难懂的）法律术语，法律用语

antidepressant ［ˌæntɪdɪˈpresnt］n. 抗抑郁药

Cymbalta 欣百达；度洛西汀

pharmaceutical ［ˌfɑːməˈsuːtɪkl］adj. 制药的；配药的；卖药的

incentive［ɪnˈsentɪv］n. 激励；刺激；鼓励

fearmongering 制造恐惧

pinpoint［ˈpɪnpɔɪnt］v. 明确指出，确定（位置或时间）

mine was unlikely to be heart-related. Just then I remembered that I'd had a glass of **carbonated** water right before going to bed—a common cause of random but pinpointed chest and abdominal pain. My own "emergency" faded away, but the state of health information online remains **dire**.

carbonated ['kɑːbəneɪtɪd] *adj.* 含二氧化碳的

dire ['daɪə(r)] *adj.* 极其严重的;危急的;极糟的

Task 1

Read the following statements and then decide whether each of them is true or false based on the information in the text. Write T for True and F for False in the blanks. Correct the false statements.

1. _____ Although the author is a doctor, he still resorted to Google because he was not sure whether to call 911.

_____

2. _____ Google provided many articles, but they were all bizarre ads.

_____

3. _____ SEO plays the trick of numbers so that Google users are attracted to click on these links.

_____

4. _____ The author recalled the days with his grandmother for some remedies for his chest pain.

_____

5. _____ The links about lung cancer scared the author to death since lung cancer often causes no pain until its later stages.

_____

6. _____ For the author, the ads are big headache because they confuse the users in term of what actions they should take.

_____

7. _____ Finally，the author's problem was solved and he was very grateful towards the Internet.

Task 2

Put the following occurrences in order of time.

_____ The author clicked on a link from WebMD，which disturbed him with some irrelevant information.

_____ The author figured out the real cause of his chest pain with the help of his university's site.

_____ The author began to Google his symptom.

_____ The author found many articles with numbers in their titles，which lead his thought to the game of algorithm.

_____ The author was woken up by a sharp chest pain.

Task 3

Retell the author's experience in your own words. Please use third person instead of first person. The following connectives are for your reference.

before	when	so	but	because
however	then	after	finally	in time

Text B

A Digital Revolution in Health
Care is Coming. Welcome It

No wonder they are called "patients". When people enter the health-care systems of rich countries today, they know what they will get: **prodding** doctors, endless tests, **baffling jargon**, rising costs and, above all, long waits. Some **stoicism** will always be needed, because health care is complex and **diligence** matters. But frustration is **boiling over**. This week three of the biggest names in American business—Amazon, Berkshire Hathaway and JPMorgan Chase—announced a new venture to provide better, cheaper health care for their employees. A fundamental problem with today's system is that patients lack knowledge and control. Access to data can **bestow** both.

The Internet already enables patients to seek online **consultations** when and where it suits them. You can take over the counter tests to analyse your blood, **sequence** your **genome** and check on the bacteria in your **gut**. Yet radical change demands a shift in emphasis, from providers to patients and from doctors to data. That shift is happening. Technologies such as the

prod [prɒd] v. 戳;捅;催促

baffle ['bæfl] v. 使困惑;难住

jargon ['dʒɑːgən] n. 行话;行业术语

stoicism ['stəʊɪsɪzəm] n. 对痛苦的默默承受或泰然处之;坚忍

diligence ['dɪlɪdʒəns] n. 勤勉;勤奋;用功

boil over (感情)爆发;失去理智

bestow [bɪ'stəʊ] v. 给予,授予

consultation [ˌkɒnsl'teɪʃn] n. 就诊

sequence ['siːkwəns] v. 测定(整套基因或分子成分的)序列

genome ['dʒiːnəʊm] n. 基因组;染色体组

gut [gʌt] n. 消化道;肠道

smartphone allow people to monitor their own health. The possibilities multiply when you add the crucial missing ingredients access to your own medical records and the ability easily to share information with those you trust. That allows you to reduce inefficiencies in your own treatment and also to provide data to help train medical algorithms. You can enhance your own care and everyone else's, too.

The doctor will be you now

Medical data may not seem like the type of **kindling** to spark a revolution. But the flow of information is likely to bear fruit in several ways. One is better diagnosis. Someone worried about their heart can now buy a **watch strap** containing a medical grade monitor that will detect **arrhythmias**. Apps are **vying** to see if they can diagnose everything from skin cancer and **concussion** to Parkinson's disease. Research is under way to see whether sweat can be analysed for **molecular biomarkers** without the need for an **invasive** blood test. Some think that changes in how quickly a person **swipes** a phone's touchscreen might signal the **onset** of cognitive problems.

A second benefit lies in the management of complex diseases. Diabetes apps can change the way patients cope, by monitoring blood-**glucose** levels and food intake, potentially reducing long-run harm such as blindness and **gangrene**. Akili Interactive, a startup, plans to seek **regulatory** approval for a video game

---

kindle ['kɪndl] v. 开始燃烧；点燃；激起（兴趣、感情等）；发展起来

watch strap ['wɒtʃ stræp] 表带

arrhythmia [ə'rɪðmɪə] n. 心律失常

vie [vaɪ] v. 激烈竞争；争夺

concussion [kən'kʌʃn] n. 脑震荡

molecular [mə'lekjələ(r)] adj. 分子的

biomarker ['baɪəʊ'mɑːkə(r)] n. 生物标志物

invasive [ɪn'veɪsɪv] adj. 侵入的

swipe [swaɪp] v. 刷

onset ['ɒnset] n. 开端，发生

glucose ['gluːkəʊs] n. 葡萄糖

gangrene ['gæŋgriːn] n. 坏疽

regulatory ['regjələtɔːri] adj. （对工商业）具有监管权的，监管的

designed to stimulate an area of the brain **implicated** in attention-deficit **hyperactivity** disorder.

Patients can also improve the efficiency of their care. Although health records are increasingly electronic, they are often still trapped in **silos**. Many contain data that machines cannot read. This can lead to delays in treatment, or worse. Many of the 250,000 deaths in America attributable to medical error each year can be traced to poorly co-ordinated care. With data at their fingertips, common standards to enable sharing and a strong incentive to get things right, patients are more likely to spot errors. On January 24th Apple laid out its plans to ask organizations to let patients use their smartphones to download their own medical records.

A final benefit of putting patients in charge stems from the generation and **aggregation** of their data. Artificial intelligence (AI) is already being trained by a unit of Alphabet, Google's present company to identify cancerous tissues and **retinal** damage. As patients' data stream from smartphones and "wearables," they will teach AIs to do evermore. Future AIs could, for instance, provide automated medical diagnosis from a description of your symptoms, spot behavioural traits that suggest you are depressed or identify if you are at special risk of cardiac disease. The aggregation of data will also make it easier for you to find other people with similar diseases and to see how they responded to various

implicate ['implikeit] v. 牵涉,涉及(某人);表明(或意指)……是起因

hyperactivity [ˌhaɪpəræk'tɪvɪtɪ] n. 多动症

silo ['saɪləʊ] n. 筒仓

aggregation [ˌægrɪ'geɪʃn] n. 聚集,集合

retinal ['retɪnl] adj. 视网膜的

treatments.

An apple a day

pitfall ['pɪtfɔːl] *n*. 危险；困难；(尤指)陷阱，隐患

huckster ['hʌkstə(r)] *n*. 强行推销的人；沿街叫卖的小贩；上门推销员

pore over 钻研；仔细阅读

disproportionately [ˌdɪsprə'pɔːʃənətlɪ] *adv*. 不成比例地

trawl [trɔːl] *v*. 查阅(资料)；搜集

transparency [træns'pærənsɪ] *n*. 透明；透明性

hale and hearty 精力充沛的；老当益壮

As with all new technologies, **pitfalls** accompany the promise. **Hucksters** will launch apps that do not work. But with regulators demanding oversight of apps that present risks to patients, users will harm only their wallets. Not everyone will want to take active control of their own health care, plenty will want the professionals to manage everything. Fine. Data can be **pored over** by those who are interested, while those who are not can opt to share data automatically with trusted providers. The benefits of new technologies often flow **disproportionately** to the rich. Those fears are mitigated by the incentives that employers, governments and insurers have to invest in cost-efficient preventive care for all. Alphabet has recently launched a firm called Cityblock Health, for example, which plans to **trawl** through patients' data to provide better care for low-income city dwellers, many of them covered by Medicaid, an insurance programme for poorer Americans.

Other risks are harder to deal with. Greater **transparency** may encourage the **hale and hearty** not to take out health insurance. They may even make it harder for the unwell to find cover. Regulations can slow that process—by requiring insurers to ignore genetic data, for example—but not stop it. Security is another worry. The more patient data are analysed in the cloud or shared with different firms，the greater the potential threat of hacking or misuse. Almost a quarter of all data **breaches** in America happen in health care. Health firms should face **stringent** penalties if they are **slapdash** about security，but it is naive to expect that breaches will ever happen.

breach [briːtʃ] *n*. (对法规等的)违背，违犯；破坏
stringent ['strɪndʒənt] *adj*. 严格的；严厉的
slapdash ['slæpdæʃ] *adj*. 仓促马虎的；潦草的

Will the benefits of making data more widely available outweigh such risks? The signs are that they will. Plenty of countries are now opening up their medical records，but few have gone as far as Sweden. It aims to give all its citizens electronic access to their medical records by 2020；over a third of Swedes have already set up accounts. Studies show that patients with such access have a better understanding of their illnesses，and that their treatment is more successful. Trials in America and Canada have produced not just happier patients but lower costs，as **clinicians fielded** fewer inquiries. That should be no surprise. No one has a greater interest in your health than you do. Trust in Doctor You.

clinician [klɪ'nɪʃn] *n*. 临床医师
field [fiːld] *v*. 接

Task 1

Helen wants to give a presentation to introduce this article to her class. Please help her complete the following mind map about the article，so that she can better understand it.

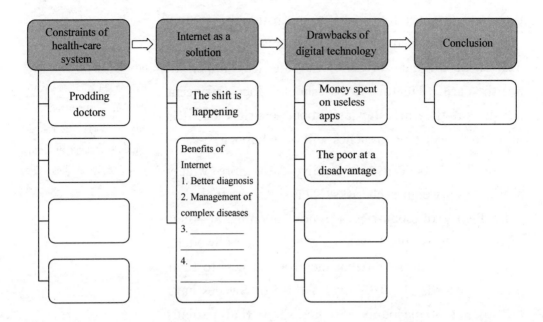

Task 2

Then，Helen makes a PPT as a visual aid to go with the presentation. Please help her prepare the following PPT slides.

Slide 1：

A digital revolution in health care is coming. Welcome it!

Overview

- Constraints of health-care system
- What is happening
- Benefits of Internet
- Drawbacks of digital technology
- Conclusion

Slide 2

What is happening now?
• _____
• _____
• _____

Slide 3

How can Internet benefit health care?
• Better diagnosis
• Better management of complex diseases
• _____
• _____

Slide 4

Challenges
• People may pay for useless apps.
• The poor are at a disadvantage.
• _____
• _____

Slide 5

Conclusion
• _____
• In Sweden ...
• In America and Canada ...

Task 3

Now Helen goes on preparing the presentation. Please write a transcript for her. The transcript should include a summary of the article.

_____

_____

_____

_____

_____

_____

_____

_____

_____

_____

_____

_____

Reading Aloud

A. 连读(liaison)3——辅辅连读、失去爆破

英语的爆破音有 3 对,/p/和/b/、/t/和/d/、/k/和/g/。失去爆破,又叫不完全爆破,就是在某些情况下,只需做出发音的准备,但并不发音,稍稍停顿后就发后面的音。

当爆破音中的任意两个相临时,前一个爆破音会失去爆破,即由相关的发音器官做好这个发音的姿势,稍做停顿后即发后面的爆破音。

The girl in the re(d) coat was on a bla(ck) bike jus(t) now.

The bi(g) bus from the fa(c)tory is full of people.

Wha(t) time does he get up every morning?

This is an ol(d) pi(c)ture of a bi(g) car.

两个相同的爆破音前后相连时,前一个音做好发音姿势,稍停顿,然后发后面的音。

The ol(d) do(c)tor has a ca(t), too.

We are going to work on a farm nex(t) Tuesday.

Would you li(k)e, ho(t) tea or bla(ck) coffee?

It's a very col(d) day, but it's a goo(d) day.

B. Read aloud after the recording.

Unlike a lot of "medical information" online, SEO i(t)self is steeped in the scientifi(c) method, which shows tha(t) this number-heavy forma(t) plays to a human co(g)nitive bias calle(d) stand-out. We notice things tha(t) stand out—like o(dd)ly precise numbers. When I was a child in Turkey, my gran(d)mother love(d) various over-the-counter remedies for maladies from the mos(t) minor to the serious, an(d) many of them containe(d) menthol. Menthol may not always have been the active ingredient, but it gave a soothing, medicinal aura to the lotions and rubs that filled her cu(p)board. Similarly, these o(dd), specific numbers add a scientific aura to the hea(d)lines.

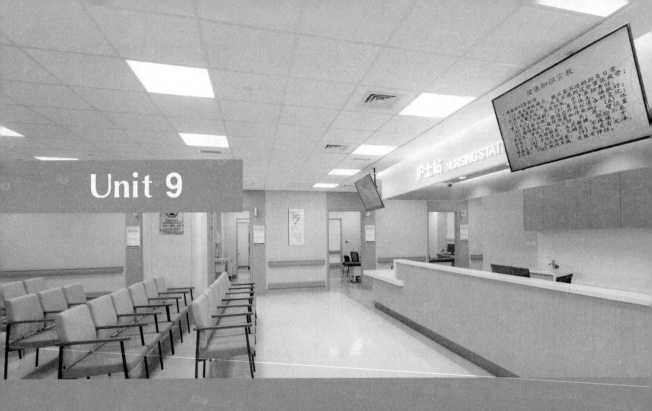

Unit 9

Upon completion of this unit, you will be able to:

- draw a mind map to clarify text's main ideas
- summarize main points of an interview
- learn the pronunciation skill of voicing

✓音视频资源
✓参考答案
✓交流探讨

Text A

Clones will Herald New Therapies, But will They Be Accepted, Asks Andy Coghlan

Meet Zhongzhong and Huahua, the world's first monkeys cloned using the technique that gave us Dolly the sheep.

The female long-tailed **macaques** represent a technical **milestone**. It should make it possible to create **customizable** and genetically uniform populations of monkeys, which could speed up treatments for diseases such as **Parkinson's**, **Alzheimer's** and cancer. But the breakthrough will inevitably raise fears that human cloning is closer than ever.

The monkeys hold such huge potential because they all inherit exactly the same genetic material, says the Chinese team that cloned them.

This would enable scientists to **tweak** genes the monkeys have that are linked to human disease, and then monitor how this alters the animals' biology, comparing it against animals that are genetically identical except for the **alterations**. It could accelerate the hunt for genes and processes that go wrong in these diseases, and ways to correct them, the team says.

herald ['herəld] v. 预示

macaque [mə'kæk] n. 猕猴

milestone ['maɪlstəʊn] n. 转折点；里程碑

customizable ['kʌstəˌmaɪzəbl] a. 可定制的；客户自定义的

Parkinson's ['pɑːkɪnsnz] n. 帕金森症

Alzheimer's ['æltshaɪməz] n. 阿尔茨海默病

tweak [twiːk] v. 稍稍调整

alteration [ˌɔːltə'reɪʃn] n. 改变；更改

mammal ['mæml] *n.* 哺乳动物

Although 23 species of **mammal** have been cloned since Dolly—including pigs，cats，dogs，rats and cattle—monkeys have，until now，proved resistant to the technique.

In 2000，researchers cloned monkeys for the first time，but did so by splitting an embryo after it had been fertilised，essentially just producing a genetically identical twin. This method can only be used to create a maximum of four identical animals.

Now，Qiang Sun at the Chinese Academy of Sciences Institute of Neuroscience in Shanghai and his colleagues have tweaked the technique used to produce Dolly to create a theoretically limitless number of clones.

somatic [səʊˈmætɪk] *adj.* 躯体的；体细胞的
nucleus['njuːkliəs] *n.* 核；细胞核

Called **somatic** cell nuclear transfer，the method involves removing the **nucleus** from a donor egg cell and replacing it with one taken out of a cell from another animal.

An electric current is used to trick the egg into thinking it has been fertilised，and it starts to develop into an early embryo. When implanted into the uterus

surrogate [ˈsʌrəgət] *adj.* 替代的；代用的

of a **surrogate** mother，the embryo will grow into a carbon copy of the animal that donated the nucleus.

Previous attempts to do this in monkeys have never progressed beyond an early embryonic stage

blastocyst [ˈblæstəʊˌsɪst] *n.* 囊胚；胚包

called a **blastocyst**.

Sun and his colleagues went further by introducing

two new ingredients to the soup of **nutrients** and growth factors that help cloned embryos grow before being placed into the surrogate. The ingredients—Messenger RNA and a compound called **trichostatin** A—awakened at least 2000 genes that are vital for various stages of embryonic development, enabling development to proceed.

nutrient ['njuːtrɪənt] n. 营养素

trichostatin [trɪ'kɒstətɪn] n. 曲古抑菌素

The team also discovered that it is easier to clone macaques if you use cells from **fetal** macaques rather than adults. Zhongzhong and Huahua were both created using cells destined to form connective tissue, extracted from an **aborted** female fetus.

fetal ['fiːtl] adj. 胎儿的

abort [ə'bɔːt] v. 使流产

Altogether, 79 embryos were implanted into 21 surrogates. The pair were thc only live births from six pregnancies. Dolly was the only success from 277 implanted embryos.

Human clones

Although attempts to perform the technique using cells taken from adult macaques also produced two live animals, both died soon after birth, and one had abnormal body development.

"For many cell types, reprogramming is more difficult for adult cells than for fetal cells," says Robert Lanza, chief scientist at the Astellas Institute for Regenerative Medicine in Massachusetts, whose team cloned human adult skin cells for the first time in 2014. "That appears to be the case here as well," he says.

hurdle［'hɜːdl］ *n*. 难关；障碍

hoax［həʊks］*n*. 骗局；恶作剧

mimic［'mɪmɪk］*v*. 模仿

replica［'replɪkə］*n*. 复制品；仿制品

This technical **hurdle** may put to rest fears often expressed after cloning successes: that it could lead to a *Never Let Me Go* scenario—the science fiction novel in which human clones are created for spare organs.

Post Dolly, the Raelian movement in California claimed it had cloned human babies. It set up a firm called Clonaid, but its efforts were dismissed as a **hoax**. "It could be a step towards human cloning, but why would you do it?" says Peter Andrews at the University of Sheffield, UK. "In terms of human biology, it's illegal to clone a human in Britain and many other countries, and I don't think anyone would rationally want to do it."

The Chinese team says its focus is to use the cloned monkeys to create better animal models of disease in order to accelerate medical therapies.

Andrews says this concept has merit, especially given the long-standing difficulties of trying to **mimic** complex diseases like Alzheimer's and Parkinson's in mice.

To date, all therapies that have treated Alzheimer's-like symptoms in mice have failed when trialed in humans. One potential reason for the repeated failure is that the Alzheimer's mouse model is not a close enough **replica** of the human version of the disease.

Now it might be possible to better model Alzheimer's in cloned monkeys by knocking out genes that have a similar role in monkeys and humans, such as one that triggers the production of beta-**amyloid plaques** that **clog up** Alzheimer's brains.

There are issues though, says Andrews. "Not least the cost of keeping **primates**, and that you'd need to breed many of them for it to be useful. You would then run into **ethical** problems—you can see why people would object."

The most recent UK assessment on the ethics of primate research, published in 2006, found "a strong scientific case for the carefully regulated use of non-human primates where there are no other means to address clearly defined questions of particular importance."

At a conference in May 2016, Mu-ming Poo of the Institute of Neuroscience in Shanghai **unveiled** the world's first genetically engineered monkey with a version of Parkinson's disease and presented ambitious plans to expand the use of monkeys to study **neurodegenerative** disease.

He made the same case in *New Scientist* shortly after, arguing that because monkeys are so closely related to us and have advanced minds and complex social networks, they will tell us much more about diseases of the brain than mice ever could.

amyloid plaque ['æmɪlɔɪd plæk]淀粉样斑块

clog up [klɒg ʌp]（使）阻塞

primate['praɪmeɪt] n. 灵长类

ethical ['eθɪkl] adj.（有关）道德的；伦理的

unveil [ˌʌn'veɪl] v.（首次）展示，介绍，推出

neurodegenerative [njʊərəʊdɪ'dʒenərətɪv] adj. 神经退化的；神经退行性的

Task 1

Draw a mind map based on what you learn from the text. Then summarize the text based on the mind map.

Task 2

Choose the one that best completes the sentence or answers the question according to the text.

1. Why does the clone of Zhongzhong and Huahua represent a technical milestone?

   A. Because human cloning is closer to us.

   B. Because it can provide potential therapy for some difficult conditions.

   C. Because people can customize monkeys as their pets.

2. "This would enable scientists to tweak genes the monkeys have that are linked to human disease." What does "tweak" mean in Sentence 1, Paragraph 4?

   A. To pull or twist suddenly.

   B. To adjust slightly.

   C. To copy.

3. In 2000，researchers cloned monkeys by _____.

   A. producing an identical twin of a fertilised embryo

   B. using the technique that created Dolly the sheep

   C. creating four identical animals

4. What's the use of electric current in cloning the monkeys?

A. To give the egg thinking ability.

B. To stimulate the egg to grow into an embryo.

C. To stimulate the embryo to grow into an animal.

5. Which is NOT the reason that some people would object to primate research?

A. High cost.

B. Ethical issue.

C. Repeated failure.

Task 3

Read the following statements and then decide whether each of them is true or false based on the text. Write T for True and F for False in the blanks.

1. _____ Zhongzhong and Huahua are the world's first cloned monkeys.

2. _____ Research on cloned monkcys could assist the identification of genes and processes that go wrong in some human diseases.

3. _____ 23 species of mammal have been cloned so far.

4. _____ The technique used to produce Dolly, Zhongzhong and Huahua is called somatic cell nuclear transfer.

5. _____ The two new ingredients added to the soup of nutrients are Messenger RNA and a compound called trichostatin A.

6. _____ It is harder to clone macaques by using cells from fetal macaques rather than adults.

7. _____ The Raelian movement's efforts were dismissed because it's illegal to clone a human.

8. _____ It's difficult to mimic some complex diseases in mice probably because the mouse model is not close enough to human.

9. _____ Mu-ming Poo's program with genetically engineered monkey has produced effective therapy for Parkinson's disease.

10. _____ Monkeys are the best candidates for human disease research because they have advanced minds and complex social networks.

Text B

cardiologist
[ˌkɑːdɪˈɒlədʒɪst] *n.* 心脏病医生；心脏病学家

Will AI Make Medicine More Human?

[**Cardiologist** Eric Topol explores how machine learning could help doctors reconnect with patients.] By Alex Orlando

Q: After 35 years as a cardiologist, what led you to transition away from patient care as a physician to focus on research and digital medicine?

A: Well, I haven't fully [transitioned] because I still see patients—I was in the clinic today. I basically just devoted more effort to the research side, but I never wanted to give up the clinical, patient care part. Because that's what it's all about, right? All the research that I'm involved in has some type of connection with patients to try and improve medicine.

Q: Why is that connection between doctor and patient so important?

A: In the clinic today, I was finishing up with a [medical] fellow who I've worked with for the last two years. One of his gifts was his ability to connect with our patients. One of the patients today was crying about him moving on and finishing his **fellowship**. That, to me, is the essence of medicine. People tend

fellowship [ˈfeləʊʃɪp] *n.* 伙伴关系；友谊；交情；研究员职位

to think I'm very high-tech and into all sorts of **gadgets**, **sensors** and AI. But having been sick [myself], I appreciate that relationship all the more. Medicine is nothing without it.

Q: You've recently talked about how medicine today is characterized by a lack of human connection between doctors and patients. For example, you've noted that electronic health records have essentially turned doctors into data technicians. How did we get to this point?

A: The **cardinal** sin was letting medicine become such a big business. The electronic health record is the single worst **abject** failure of modern medicine, because it was set up for business purposes—for **billing**—only, without any regard for what would benefit doctors, patients or any other clinicians. That's one big part of it.

The other is the unchecked growth of **administrative personnel**, with a ratio of approximately 10 to 1 compared with those who actually take care of patients. All of this was to increase productivity. Unfortunately, over the course of decades, medicine lost its way.

Q: Do patients have any power in today's medical **landscape**, or does technology always work against their interests?

A: There's **tension** here, because some things are promoting [patients'] **empowerment**, like the ability to

---

gadget['gædʒɪt] *n.* 小器具;小装置

sensor ['sensə(r)] *n.* 传感器,敏感元件,探测设备

cardinal ['kɑːdɪnl] *adj.* 最重要的;基本的

abject ['æbdʒekt] *adj.* 悲惨绝望的;凄惨的

billing ['bɪlɪŋ] *n.* 营业额

administrative personnel [əd'mɪnɪstrətɪv ˌpɜːsə'nel] (总称)行政人员

landscape ['lændskeɪp] *n.* 形势;情形

tension ['tenʃn] *n.* 矛盾;对立

empowerment [ɪm'paʊəmənt] *n.* 授权

generate their own data. One example is an Apple Watch, where they could get their heart rhythm detected if it's abnormal. Or, in the UK, you can get **urinary tract** infections diagnosed with an AI kit. Or you can get your child's ear infection diagnosed without a doctor, through a smartphone. And [soon it will be possible to diagnose] **lesions**, **rashes** or cancer of the skin through a picture and an algorithm. There are many different ways in which [patient] empowerment is **getting off the ground**. And it's doctorless, with sensors and cameras that will lead to an algorithmic interpretation that's accurate—without the need to connect with a doctor.

But at the same time, we have this **sparse** data access and lack of control by the individual, who should be the **rightful** owner [of their own medical data].

Q: Let's talk about patient data. Some types of artificial intelligence, like machine learning algorithms that interpret imaging scans, take place behind the curtain, completely invisible to patients. Should they know when—and how—their data is going to be used?

A: AI has crept into people's lives in so many ways—whether it's a recommendation for a song, an Amazon purchase or a word [that] autocorrects. All of these things are happening. So this algorithmic invisibility got **embedded** in our lives. It's one thing to have an autocorrect; it's another thing to have a

Glossary:

urinary tract ['jʊərɪnəri trækt] 泌尿道;泌尿管;尿路

lesion ['liːʒn] n. (因伤病导致皮肤或器官的)损伤,损害

rash [ræʃ] n. 皮疹;疹

get off the ground 起飞;顺利开始

sparse [spɑːs] adj. 稀少的

rightful ['raɪtfl] adj. 正确的;公正的;合法的

embed [ɪm'bed] v. 把……牢牢地嵌入

medical issue. I think we need to take a step back and **partition** the normal, daily-life things that aren't serious matters versus the algorithms that will be part of one's medical diagnostics and treatments.

partition [pɑːˈtɪʃn] *v.* 分割；使分裂

Q: How concerned are you about racial bias in health care, including AI? For instance, a 2019 study in *Science* found that a widely used algorithm was racially biased. The algorithm was intended to help hospitals predict which patients might benefit from additional treatment, based on their previous "cost of care," or their past medical expenses. But it assigned the same level of "risk" to sicker black patients as it did to healthier white patients. How can AI become biased?

A: Algorithms don't know about bias; it's about the humans that are putting the data in. Here, the big mistake was that the [developers] assumed that if you had a lower cost of care in the database, that meant you were healthier. But, no, it could mean that you just don't have access to care. As it turned out, when the [researchers] looked at the data, they realized that many of the people who had low cost of care were black people who had no or little access. It had nothing to do with the algorithm. What we have is human bias, and we then blame it on the machines.

Q: What about mental illness—can AI help there?

A: This is one of the most exciting new directions that we have. Because mental health problems,

across the board 影响全体地；全面地

understaffed
[ˌʌndəˈstɑːft] *adj*. 人员不足；人手太少

counselor [ˈkaʊns(ə)lə]
n. 顾问

psychiatrist [saɪˈkaɪətrɪst]
n. 精神病学家；精神科医生

parameter [pəˈræmɪtə(r)]
n. 决定因素

avatar [ˈævətɑː(r)] *n*. 化身

replicate [ˈreplɪkeɪt] *v*. 复制；(精确地)仿制；再造

reconcile [ˈrekənsaɪl] *v*. 调和；妥协

surveillance [sɜːˈveɪləns]
n. 监视

particularly depression but all **across the board**, are so important. They're also **understaffed** in terms of capable **counselors**, psychologists, **psychiatrists** and mental health professionals in general. So the ability to quantify, in real time, a person's state of mind is an extraordinary new development. Whether that's how you strike a keyboard, the intonation of your speech, your breathing or all of the other **parameters** that can be assessed passively, without any effort. There are many different ways to capture that data. Now, we can quantify that. We've never been able to do that—it was all subjective, like, "Are you feeling blue?"

The other [development] was the realization that people are entirely comfortable talking to [AI] **avatars**. They don't have to talk to a human. In fact, they'd prefer to disclose their innermost secrets to an avatar. That still, to me, is shocking, but it's been **replicated** with multiple studies now.

The field using AI in mental health care, while it's still very underdeveloped and early, is one of the greatest opportunities going forward. Because there's a terrible mismatch of the burden of mental health and the field's ability to support people. I think the promise here is quite extraordinary. It's using technology to enhance human mental health, which never tends to get the same respect as physical health.

Q: How do you **reconcile** your optimism with AI's darker side, like the potential for **surveillance** and data hacking?

A: Well, I'm an optimistic person; I always have been. My wife always **chides** me about that. ... [But] I'm aware of where things can go wrong—everything from a **nefarious** attack on an algorithm to a plain software **glitch** that we're all too familiar with. And bias making **inequities** worse. All sorts of **disruptive**, **dystopian** things.

Awareness of that is one part of the story. Another, interestingly, is that AI can make things better or worse across the board. It can make inequities worse, or it can make them better; it can make bias worse or it could improve it. Any way you look, you can say that it's a two-edged sword. It's very powerful and it could make a lot of these things better or worse. Only time will tell, and we're in the very early stages, for sure.

Q: Why did you become so invested in exploring how AI might bring humanity back to health care?

A: We're in a desperate state, and we need to acknowledge the lack of human connection and empathy [in medicine]. It's the loss of the "care" in health care. We may be looking at our best potential solution for multiple generations to come. This is more attractive, at least from its potential, than anything I've seen throughout my 35 years. I'm an old dog, and I've seen a lot, but never anything like this.

I do think it's going to take a lot of work and a lot

chide [tʃaɪd] v. 批评；指责；责备

nefarious [nɪˈfeərɪəs] adj. 罪恶的；不道德的

glitch [glɪtʃ] n. 小故障；小毛病；小差错

inequity [ɪnˈekwəti] n. 不公正的事；不公正；不公平

disruptive [dɪsˈrʌptɪv] adj. 引起混乱的；扰乱性的；破坏性的

dystopian [dɪsˈtəʊpɪən] adj. 反乌托邦的

validation [ˌvælɪˈdeɪʃən] *n.* 验证；确认；证实；核实

of **validation**. When you have something as powerful as this, and if you do it right, you can get medicine back on track to the way it was 40 years ago—at that time, it was a whole different model. It was a very close, trusted relationship when you were with the doctor. And you knew that when you were sick, there was somebody there who had your back; who really cared for you, had time for you and wasn't looking at a computer screen. We could get that back. That's exciting.

Q: How far are we from that reality?

A: Because of my optimism, I tend to always guess too short of a time. And then I look at my grandchildren, who are ages 5 and 2. And I'm just hoping that, realistically, by the time they get older, it'll have restored medicine. But it's going to take a while. It's not going to happen in one fell **swoop**, either. But I'm hoping that we'll see the beginning of that in the next five years. And **billboards**, instead of **touting** that the health system is the best in the country, will instead say, "We give our patients time. We give our doctors and nurses time with patients." If we start seeing competitiveness among health systems for the gift of time, that will be the beginning of this "back to the future" story.

swoop [swuːp] *n.* 突然行动

billboard [ˈbɪlbɔːd] *n.* （大幅）广告牌

tout [taʊt] *v.* 标榜；吹捧；吹嘘

Task 1

Choose the one that best completes the sentence or answers the question according to the text.

1. Which of the following statements is true about Eric Topol?

   A. He transitioned away from patient care as physician to focus on research.

   B. He transitioned away from patient care as physician to focus on AI.

   C. He has been working as a cardiologist for 35 years and will go on being one.

2. Why does Dr Topol mention a fellow he worked with for the last two years?

   A. To acknowledge his work in the clinic.

   B. To show the importance of doctor-patient connection.

   C. To show regret about the colleague's leaving.

3. Dr Topol agrees with the following statements EXCEPT _____.

   A. that electronic health records is dehumanizing medicine

   B. that pursuit of commercial profit is disrupting modern medicine

   C. that today's medical institutions are overstaffed

4. Which of the following statements is true according to Eric Topol?

   A. Technology empowers patients to diagnose their diseases so that doctors are less needed.

   B. Technology empowers patients so that they can generate their own data.

   C. Technology empowers patients so that they can control their medical data.

5. When Dr Topol answers the fifth question, he says "It's one thing to have an autocorrect; it's another thing to have a medical issue." What does this sentence mean?

   A. It means different technologies are used in these two.

   B. It means the former is less invisible than the latter.

   C. It means the latter is more critical than the former.

6. Who is to blame in the racial bias black patients suffer?

A. AI technology.

B. Algorithms.

C. Human mistake.

7. How does AI enhance human mental health?

A. By quantifying people's mental condition.

B. By asking patients questions like "Are you feeling blue?"

C. By provide patients avatars as their company.

8. Why is Dr Topol so enthusiastic about AI research?

A. Because AI is a two-edged sword.

B. Because we're in the early stages of AI research.

C. Because AI can bring about unprecedented change to medicine.

9. What does Dr Topol hope to see in five years?

A. AI would get medicine back on track to the way it was 40 years ago.

B. New technology would begin to restore ideal doctor-patient relationship.

C. Health systems would advertise time as their superiority.

Task 2

Complete the following table with key words, summarized questions and answers in each turn of the interview.

Turn of interview	Key words	Concise questions	Concise answers
1st turn	AI research, physician	What led Dr Topol to transition from the job of physician to AI research?	He doesn't transition because he is doing both.
2nd turn	doctor-patient connection	Why is doctor-patient connection important?	

（Continue）

Turn of interview	Key words	Concise questions	Concise answers
3rd turn	dehumanization		1. 2.
4th turn			
5th turn			
6th turn			
7th turn			1. 2. 3.
8th turn			
9th turn			
10th turn			

Task 3

Based on the text, how do you answer the question in the title: How could machine learning help doctors reconnect with patients?

Reading Aloud

A. 浊化(voicing)

英语中的清辅音浊化指清辅音在发音时发与其相对应的浊辅音的音，如清辅音/p/浊化成/b/，/t/浊化成/d/，/k/浊化成/g/，/tr/浊化成/dr/。这只是一种发音现象，不是规律。

清辅音浊化需具备的条件：

(1) 清辅音/p/、/t/、/k/、/r/紧接在/s/后；

(2) 清辅音/p/、/t/、/k/、/tr/后紧接元音；

(3) 清辅音/p/、/t/、/k/、/t/和/s/在同一音节，且该音节为重读或次重读音节。

(4) 结构：同一重读或次重读音节中，/s/ + /p/、/t/、/k/、/tr/ + 元音，读音浊化为/s/ + /b/、/d/、/g/、/dr/ + 元音，书写不变。

清辅音浊化举例：

(1) /p/浊化为/b/：speak[sbiːk]，split [sblɪt]

(2) /t/浊化为/d/：stand[sdand]，student ['sdjuːdnt]

(3) /k/浊化为/g/：school[sguːl]，scheme [sgiːm]

(4) /tr/浊化为/dr/：street [sdriːt]，strike [sdraɪk]

rest [rest]不浊化，因为辅音/t/后无元音，display[dɪ'spleɪ]和 as/tro/nau/ti/cal [ˌæstrə'nɔtɪkəl]不浊化，因为/s/和/tr/不在同一音节，spe/ci/fic[spə'sɪfɪk]、mon/ster ['mɒnstə]、mi/ni/ster['mɪnɪstər]中，/s/和其后清辅音虽在同一音节，但不是重读或次重读音节。

在美音中，/t/在单词的中间常被浊化成/d/。如：writer 和 rider，letter 和 ladder，听起来发音几乎没有区别。

B. Read aloud after the recording.

1. Researchers cloned monkeys for the first time, but did so by <u>splitting</u> an embryo after it had been fertilized.

2. An electric current is used to trick the egg into thinking it has been

fertilized, and it <u>starts</u> to develop into an early embryo.

3. Previous attempts to do this in monkeys have never progressed beyond an early embryonic <u>stage</u> called a blastocyst.

4. It could lead to a *Never Let Me Go* scenario—the science fiction novel in which human clones are created for <u>spare</u> organs.

5. Andrews says this concept has merit, especially given the long-<u>standing</u> difficulties of trying to mimic complex diseases like Alzheimer's and Parkinson's in mice.

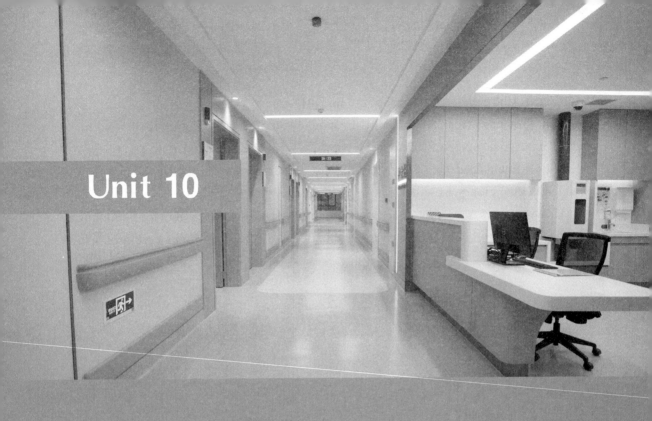

Unit 10

Upon completion of this unit，you will be able to：

- summarize the key differences between two cases
- retell two cases in contrast
- summarize the key points in an argument
- retell the story with the help of connectives given
- learn the pronunciation skill of pausing

✓音视频资源
✓参考答案
✓交流探讨

Text A

Euthanasia and a Final Gift

[Should it be easier for the terminally ill to donate organs?]

By Claudia Wallis

The first time Fred Gillis noticed something was wrong he was on the ice, holding his hockey stick but somehow unable to shoot the **puck**. Was middle age catching up with him, or was it something more serious? Over the following months Gillis's arms continued to weaken. Soon it took two hands to brush his teeth, and he couldn't lift a plate to clear the dinner table. Gillis was 52 in 2015 when he got the diagnosis he dreaded most: **amyotrophic lateral sclerosis**（**ALS**）, the deadly **motor neuron** disorder sometimes called Lou Gehrig's disease. "Fred had a co-worker whose husband had ALS," recalls his widow, Lana Gregoire. "He wanted to die from anything but that."

Both Gillis and Gregoire worked in Canadian law enforcement. They were **pragmatic**, realistic and familiar with death. "We used these three words," she says. "You have to accept, then you have to adapt and then you have to be at peace." A public servant to the

euthanasia [ˌjuːθəˈneɪzɪə] n. 安乐死

puck [pʌk] n.（冰球运动使用的）冰球

amyotrophic   lateral sclerosis（ALS）肌萎缩性侧束硬化症

motor   neuron [ˌməʊtə ˈnjʊərɒn] n. 运动神经元

pragmatic [præɡˈmætɪk] adj. 讲求实效的；务实的

core，Gillis found peace by participating in and raising money for ALS research. But a new Canadian law gave him an unexpected opportunity to make his dying days even more meaningful. In June 2016 Canada became the sixth country in the world to permit medical assistance in dying （MAID） to end intolerable suffering for terminally ill patients，and organ donation organizations had begun to develop guidelines that would allow people choosing MAID to also make a plan to donate their organs for **transplant**.

transplant ［træns'plɑːnt］
n.（器官等的）移植；移植器官

Gillis had not been a fan of the euthanasia law，but when he learned he could combine MAID with a plan to donate organs，"he was **ecstatic**," Gregoire says. "His attitude was，'ALS，you can't take this away. We're going to give life to other people.'"

ecstatic ［ɪk'stætɪk］ *adj*.
狂喜的；热情极高的

Combining euthanasia with organ donation may sound logical，but it is **ethically fraught** and not widely done. In 2017 the Netherlands became the first country to publish clinical guidelines for the practice. It established a key ethical principle：the decision to seek medical assistance in dying must precede and be separate from the organ donation plan，so that patients make their **fateful** choice without feeling pressure to donate. In Canada，each province has its own organ donation organization，and only some are working with MAID patients. The experience of three such organizations with the first 30 MAID donors was reported in a recent issue of the *New England Journal of Medicine*. In Canada，nearly two thirds of people

ethically［'eθɪklɪ］ *adv*. 道德上地；伦理上地
fraught［frɔːt］ *adj*. 忧虑的；担心的

fateful［'feɪtfl］ *adj*. 对未来有重大（负面）影响的

who qualify for MAID have active cancer and are therefore **ineligible** to donate organs; others may be too elderly. The report looked at 56 patients who were deemed eligible, 30 of whom went on to donate a total of 74 lifesaving organs.

"The feedback we heard from these patients is that they want to hear about the opportunity and make that decision themselves," says Andrew Healey, chief medical officer at the Trillium Gift of Life Network in Ontario and a co-author of the report. "People feel comfortable saying yes, and people feel comfortable saying no." In other countries that permit euthanasia, he says, the patient typically must be the one to **broach** the idea of donation.

In the US, MAID is permitted in nine states and Washington, D.C., but has not been combined with organ donation. Of course, anyone with a terminal disease can designate their organs for donation, but such plans often fail because death comes too slowly, says Joshua Mezrich, a transplant surgeon at the University of Wisconsin School of Medicine and Public Health. Even if the patient is on life support and a decision is made to pull the plug, about 30 percent of the time the organs become **nonviable** as blood pressure drops and **circulation grinds to a halt**. Mezrich has written movingly about an ALS patient named Wayne Bender who **fervently** wished to donate a kidney while he was still alive and hoped to donate more organs after death. In the end, he could do neither. The

ineligible [ɪnˈelɪdʒəbl]
adj. 不合格的;不符合资格的

broach[brəʊtʃ] *v.* 开始谈论,引入(尤指令人尴尬或有异议的话题)

nonviable [nɒnˈvaɪəbl]
a. 不能生活的;不能(无力)存活的
circulation [ˌsɜːkjəˈleɪʃn]
n. 血液循环
grind to a halt 逐渐停止
fervently[ˈfɜːvəntlɪ] *adv.* 热烈地;热情地;强烈地

veto ['vi:təʊ] *n*. 反对；否定

kidney plan was **veto** by the hospital's legal experts out of concern that Bender might die as a result of donation—an event that would violate the Dead Donor Rule，a cardinal principle of organ transplantation. And Bender died too slowly for his organs to be taken after death.

imminent ['ɪmɪnənt] *adj*. 即将发生的；临近的

murky ['mɜːki] *adj*. 隐晦的；含糊的

intravenous [ˌɪntrə'vi:nəs] *adj*. 注入静脉的；静脉内

Some experts have proposed a concept called **imminent** death donation that would allow the kind of kidney donation Bender had in mind，but its moral and legal status remain **murky**. Interestingly，donation works well after MAID because patients die quickly from the **intravenous** euthanasia drugs. Fred Gillis was able to donate two kidneys，his lungs and his liver when he died in April 2018. "He knew he was giving life，and that's all that mattered，" Gregoire says. She and their three kids were by his side and toasted him that evening—at a hockey bar. "We knew he would like that."

Task 1

Compare the story of Fred Gillis and Wayne Bender by completing the following table.

		Fred Gillis	Wayne Bender
Similarities	Disease		
	Decision		
Differences	Nationality		
	Policy		
	Result		
	Detailed reason		

Task 2

Tell the story of Fred Gillis and Wayne Bender based on the table in Task 1.

Task 3

Answer the following questions.

1. What does "final gift" in the title mean?

2. How did Fred Gillis's symptom develop?

3. What cause Fred Gillis to change his attitude toward euthanasia?

4. Why is combining euthanasia with organ donation not widely done in most countries?

5. How do you answer the question in the title: Should it be easier for the terminally ill to donate organs?

Text B

How Doctors Determine the Moment of Death?

omen ['əumən] *n*. 预兆；前兆；征兆

beeper ['biːpə(r)] *n*. 寻呼机；传呼机

It was a bad **omen** when my **beeper** went off one morning at 6：10 as I warmed up my car in the garage. Trey，my senior ICU fellow，asked me to meet him in the emergency room to save time on an admission. "A guy fell on Comm Ave this morning and cracked his head." He informed me when I rang him back. "He's got a big **subdural**，but the neurosurgeons don't want him because he may be too far gone."

subdural [sʌb'djuər(ə)l] *adj*. 硬脑膜下；硬膜下；硬膜下的

When I arrived at the Emergency Department，I found the poor guy—a very thin，**elfin**-looking man，with **pallid** skin and short，**whitish**，sparse hair—breathing on a ventilator.

elfin ['elfɪn] *n*. 精灵 *adj*. 小巧玲珑的

pallid ['pælɪd] *adj*. (尤指因病)苍白的

whitish ['waɪtɪʃ] *adj*. 发白的；稍白的

Knowing when someone's alive and knowing when someone's dead：it's one of the most important jobs that doctors do. If we can't do that，we can't do anything.

apnea [æp'nɪə] *n*. 呼吸暂停；窒息

brainstem ['breɪnstem] *n*. 脑干

forewarn [fɔː'wɔːn] *v*. 预先警告；事先告诫

The person must have an **apnea** test. Then you can prove to yourself that the whole brain，including the **brainstem**，is gone. Just remember，when you take a patient off a ventilator，either for an apnea test or after a declaration of death，make sure that family members are out of sight，and **forewarn** the nurses.

Many brain dead patients, once the ventilator is removed, exhibit the so-called **Lazarus sign**, where their arms **spontaneously contract** and their hands come up to their chest as though they're grasping for the **endotracheal tube**. It's **creepy** no matter how many times you've seen it.

This test is the big one. The object is to see whether the patient will breathe on his own. We sent 100 percent oxygen through Mike Kavanagh's lungs for two minutes, enough to sustain his heart and blood pressure without a ventilator for the next ten minutes, then shut off the ventilator.

Silence. I could hear my pocket watch ticking. As Trey and I watched closely, we could see a few arching movements in Mike's back, definitely not Lazarus sign, but something not entirely **compatible** with brain death. We waited. I felt air moving almost **imperceptibly** in and out of the ventilator tube. Was he breathing? It was important to be sure.

Ten minutes were up, and the result was conclusive. Mike Kavanagh had failed the apnea test.

"That's a **wrap**," Trey said, snapping off his gloves.

"Is it? If he's dead, in what sense is he dead?"

"In the dead sense," Trey replied.

"Well, his brain may be dead, but his other organs are alive. They can be transplanted."

Lazarus sign 拉撒路现象

spontaneously [spɒnˈteɪnɪəslɪ] *adv.* 自发；自动

contract [ˈkɒntrækt; kənˈtrækt] *n./v.* (使)收缩

endotracheal tube [ˌendəʊˈtreɪkɪəl tjuːb] 气管导管

creepy [ˈkriːpɪ] *adj.* 令人毛骨悚然的；令人不寒而栗的

compatible [kəmˈpætəbl] *adj.* 兼容的；可共存的

imperceptibly [ˌɪmpəˈseptəblɪ] *adv.* 极微地；微细地；察觉不到地

wrap [ræp] *n.* (拍摄电影时)完成拍摄，停机

"But they're just organs. Organs can be sustained, even grown outside of a body, independent of a body."

gash [gæʃ] *n.* 深长的切口（或伤口、划伤）

lymph node ['lɪmf nəʊd] 淋巴结

on automatic pilot 轻车熟路；习惯性地做

"The **gash** on his neck where the transplant surgeon cuts out a **lymph node** would heal."

"Those are just cells," Trey countered. "They're **on automatic pilot**. You provide them with blood, they keep going, but there's nothing meaningful going on."

term [tɜːm] *n.* 到期，期满

"But if Mike Kavanagh were a pregnant woman," I said, "we could keep him alive in order to bring the baby to **term**. What could be more meaningful than that? My point is that we just engaged in an operational decision, not a biological one. The end result is still correct, but we shouldn't pat ourselves on the back and say that we have come to an **ontological** certainty. We need to be honest about what we're doing. His brain may be dead, but the rest of him is not dead, and we can use the rest of him. I have no problem with what we're doing, but we should think it through more carefully."

ontological [ˌɒntəˈlɒdʒɪkl] *adj.* 本体论的

Trey paused, and said, "And that's what we just did, right?"

"You're not buying it, are you?"

"No," he replied.

death certificate ['deθ səˈtɪfɪkət] 死亡证明书

unambiguous [ˌʌnæmˈbɪɡjʊəs] *adj.* 意思清楚的；明确的

Trey and I knew very well what would happen when I signed the **death certificate**. Brain death is a firm, **unambiguous**, and operationally solid determination, an absolute point of no return for the brain. Any two competent neurologists or neurosurgeons who examine a brain-dead patient will come to the same conclusion, just as we had: this entire brain will never recover, and all the king's horses and men can't do a damn thing about it.

The problem is the word dead. It **muddies** the important issue, as does diagnosis. Brain death is not a diagnosis—a word that suggests probability—but rather a determination. A diagnosis raises the **specter** of **false positives**, of **fallibility**, of someone being buried alive. That can only happen if someone does the test incorrectly, and we hadn't.

"Look, Trey," I said, "it's fine to have an operational definition to work with. We couldn't get through the day without that. But you are in a position, because you are a doctor of the brain, to think about these things more broadly, and you should, because if you don't, nobody will."

Trey was satisfied with "merely dead," as was the Presidential Commission, the **Commonwealth** of Massachusetts, and the **Vatican**. I'm not entirely sure.

muddy ['mʌdɪ] v. 使变得泥泞;使浑浊

specter ['spektə(r)] n. 恐惧;恐慌;忧虑;鬼;幽灵
false positive [fɔːls'pɒzətɪv] 假阳性
fallibility [ˌfælə'bɪləti] n. 不可靠性

Commonwealth ['kɒmənwelθ] 联邦
Vatican ['vætɪkən] n. 梵蒂冈(罗马天主教教廷)

Task 1

There is some disagreement between the author and Doctor Trey about whether the patient was dead. What are these contradictions? Find them and fill in the following table.

Author's arguments	Doctor Trey's arguments
The patient was not dead.	

Task 2

1. Complete the following flow chart about the story.

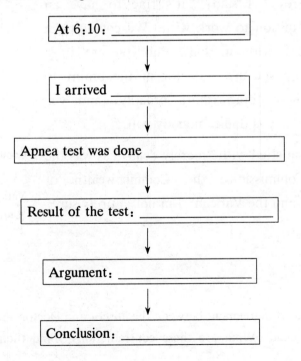

At 6:10: _____

I arrived _____

Apnea test was done _____

Result of the test: _____

Argument: _____

Conclusion: _____

Task 3

Choose the appropriate connectives from the box and retell the story based on the chart. (You don't have to use all of the connectives.)

when	so	immediately	because
however	then	after	eventually

Reading Aloud

A. 停顿(pause)

如何把握英语朗读的节奏与停顿?

意群(sense-group):一个句子可根据意思和语法结构分成若干小段,每一小段称之为一个意群。意群是句子内部有相对完整意义的一组词,可以是一个词、一个词组或短语,也可以是并列句的一个分句或复合句的一个主句、从句等等,我们可用"/"来划分句子的意群。

停顿(pause):在一个较长的句子中,如果按意群来读,意群之间稍加停顿,就可以让听者听清我们语流中的意群和句子,体现出英语所特有的节奏和韵律,但是在一个意群中不可停顿。

如:Afterschool,/my classmates and I/are going to play basketball.

Early to bed /and early to rise /makes a man /healthy, happy, and wise.

We must do /what we know is right,/and do it /with all our might.

A child begins to speak /the moment he opens his lips / to utter any acknowledged sound.

B. Read aloud after the recording.

The first time Fred Gillis noticed something was wrong /he was on the ice, /holding his hockey stick /but somehow unable to shoot the puck. /Was middle age catching up with him, /or was it something more serious? /Over the following months /Gillis's arms continued to weaken. /Soon it took two hands /to brush his teeth, /and he couldn't lift a plate /to clear the dinner table. /Gillis was 52 in 2015 /when he got the diagnosis he dreaded most:/amyotrophic lateral sclerosis (ALS), /the deadly motor neuron disorder /sometimes called Lou Gehrig's disease. /"Fred had a co-worker /whose husband had ALS," /recalls his widow, /Lana Gregoire. /"He wanted to die /from anything but that."

Glossary

pelvic *adj*. 靠近骨盆的；骨盆的　　　　6A

perfunctorily *adv*. 敷衍地；马马虎虎　　3A

persevere *v*. 坚持；孜孜以求　　　　　　3A

personnel *n*.（组织或军队中的）全体人员，

　　职员　　　　　　　　　　　　　　4A

petroleum *n*. 石油；原油　　　　　　　7B

pharmaceutical *adj*. 制药的；配药的；

　　卖药的　　　　　　　　　　　　　8A

physician *n*. 医师；（尤指）内科医生　2A

physiology *n*. 生理学　　　　　　　　1B

physiotherapy *n*. 理疗；物理治疗　　　6A

pick on 跟……找碴；故意刁难　　　　　1A

pinpoint *v*. 明确指出，确定（位置或时间）8A

pipe up 开始（大声）讲话　　　　　　　6A

pitfall *n*. 危险；困难；（尤指）陷阱，隐患　8B

placement *n*. 安置，放置　　　　　　8A

plasticity *n*. 可塑性　　　　　　　　1B

plod *v*. 艰难地行走；吃力地行进　　　7B

poignant *adj*. 令人沉痛的；悲惨的；酸楚的　1B

polycystic ovary syndrome 多囊卵巢综合征 6A

pore *n*.（皮肤上的）毛孔　　　　　　7B

pore over 钻研；仔细阅读　　　　　　8B

pragmatic *adj*. 讲求实效的；务实的　10A

predator *n*. 捕食性动物；掠夺者　　　5A

predominantly *adv*. 主要地；多数情况下　6B

preferential *adj*. 优先的；优惠的；优待的　3A

prescription *n*. 处方；药方　　　　　2B

pretzel *n*. 椒盐卷饼　　　　　　　　7A

primary sclerosing cholangitis 原发性

　　硬化性胆管炎　　　　　　　　　6A

primate *n*. 灵长类　　　　　　　　　9A

prioritize *v*. 按重要性排列；划分优先顺序；

　　优先处理　　　　　　　　　　　2A

prodrome *n*. 前驱症状；先兆　　　　　1A

prod *v*. 戳；捅；催促　　　　　　　　8B

professionalism *n*. 专业水平；专业素质　1A

pro-inflammatory *adj*. 促炎性的；致发炎的；

　　促发炎的　　　　　　　　　　　7B

prominent *adj*. 显眼的；显著的；突出的　7A

psychiatrist *n*. 精神病学家；精神科医生　9B

puck *n*.（冰球运动使用的）冰球　　　10A

quackery *n*. 江湖医术；庸医行径　　　8A

quarantine *v*./*n*.（对动物或人）进行检疫，

　　隔离　　　　　　　　　　　　　4A

quiver *v*. 轻微颤动；抖动　　　　　　1A

radical *adj*. 根本的；彻底的；完全的　7A

rally *v*. 召集；集合　　　　　　　　　5A

rash *n*. 皮疹；疹　　　　　　　　　　9B

reception *n*. 接待处；接待区　　　　　4B

receptor *n*. 感受器；受体　　　　　　7B

reconcile *v*. 调和；妥协　　　　　　　9B

refire *v*. 再点燃　　　　　　　　　　7B

regale *v*.（以故事或笑话）极力取悦　　3A

regenerate *v*. 再生；使再生　　　　　7B

regulate *v*. 约束，控制　　　　　　　5B

regulatory *adj*.（对工商业）具有监管权的，

　　监管的　　　　　　　　　　　　8B

replenish *v*. 补充　　　　　　　　　7B

replica *n*. 复制品；仿制品　　　　　　9A

replicate *v*. 复制；（精确地）仿制；再造　9B

rep *n*. 推销员；销售代表　　　　　　3A

reproductive *adj*. 生殖的；繁殖的　　5B

residency *n*. 住院医生实习期　　　　　3A

resilience *n*. 快速恢复的能力；适应力；

　　还原能力；弹力　　　　　　　　7A

resonance *n*. 共鸣；共振　　　　　　1B

retinal *adj*. 视网膜的　　　　　　　　8B